THE DEVELOPMENT OF A NEW TRIPHASIC ORAL CONTRACEPTIVE

THE DEVELOPMENT OF A NEW TRIPHASIC ORAL CONTRACEPTIVE

The Proceedings of a Special Symposium held at the 10th World Congress on Fertility and Sterility, Madrid, July 1980

Co-ordinating Editors:
J. Cortés-Prieto and A. Campos-da-Paz

Edited by R. B. Greenblatt

MTP PRESS LIMITED
International Medical Publishers

Published by
MTP Press Limited
Falcon House
Lancaster, England

Softcover reprint of the hardcover 1st edition 1984

First published 1984

British Library Cataloguing in Publication Data

Ratnesar, P.
Problems in otolaryngolgy. – (Problems in practice series)
i. Otolaryngology
I.Title II.Series
616.2'2 RF46

ISBN-13: 978-94-011-6668-3 e-ISBN-13: 978-94-011-6666-9
DOI: 10.1007/978-94-011-6666-9

Frome and London

Contents

List of Contributors

H. H. Allen
Clinical Professor,
Department of Obstetrics and Gynaecology,
University of Western Ontario,
London,
Canada

M. Briggs
Dean of Science,
Professor of Biology,
Deakin University,
Victoria 3217,
Australia

Maxine Briggs
Geelong Hospital,
Victoria 3220,
Australia

L. Fåhreus
MD,
Department of Obstetrics and Gynaecology,
University Hospital,
Linköping,
Sweden

R. B. Greenblatt
Professor Emeritus, Endocrinology,
Medical College of Georgia,
Augusta,
Georgia 30912,
USA

U. Lachnit-Fixson
Head of the Department of Clinical Endocrinology,
Schering AG,
D-1000 Berlin 65,
West Germany

U. Larsson-Cohn
Professor,
Department of Obstetrics and Gynaecology,
University Hospital,
Linköping,
Sweden

E. R. Plunkett
Department of Obstetrics and Gynaecology,
University of Western Ontario,
London,
Canada

W. H. F. Schneider
Professor,
First Department of Obstetrics and Gynaecology,
University of Vienna,
A-1090 Vienna,
Austria

R. P. Smith
Department of Obstetrics and Gynaecology,
University of Western Ontario,
London,
Canada

J. Spona
Professor,
Endocrine Research Unit,
First Department of Obstetrics and Gynaecology,
University of Vienna,
A-1090 Vienna,
Austria

G. Virginia Upton
Associate Director Clinical Research,
Wyeth International Limited,
P.O. Box 8616,
Philadelphia,
PA 19101,
USA

L. Wallentin
Professor,
Department of Internal Medicine,
University Hospital,
Linköping,
Sweden

G. Zador
Professor,
Kabi AB,
Stockholm,
Sweden

Editorial note

The new triphasic oral contraceptive referred to throughout this text is currently manufactured and marketed by

Schering AG Berlin Bergkamen
under the registered trade names of:
Triquilar® Logynon®

Wyeth International Limited
under the registered trade name of:
Trinordiol®

This product is also referred to as SH B 264 AB and WL-49(50) in certain reports

1
A retrospective view of oral contraceptives

R. B. GREENBLATT

Ever since man became aware of the relationship between coitus and pregnancy, he has searched for some method – mechanical, medicinal, magical – which would prevent conception or limit the number of progeny. A variety of contraceptive measures has been in vogue: coitus interruptus, vaginal jellies and foams, diaphragms, condoms, and the rhythm method. These modalities, however, leave much to be desired, from the point of view of both aesthetics and individual acceptability and safety.

The advent of hormonal control of conception fired the imagination of the medical world. The promise of almost 100% security is indeed true and millions of women have found an answer to their needs without jeopardizing the sexual act. The limitation of offspring for whatever reason – ill health, economics, planned spacing of childbirth, or personal reasons – may now be carried out with ease, convenience and dignity. However, the risks and hazards of the Pill gradually presented and from time to time alarms have been sounded about the safety of oral contraceptives. The cogent reason for this symposium on advances in hormonal contraception is the prospect of minimizing untoward effects by an improved formulation of the Pill.

THE BIRTH OF THE PILL

The absence of ovulation during the period of ascendancy of the corpus luteum was known for almost 50 years before Makepeace demonstrated in 1937 that progesterone is an effective inhibitor of copulation-induced ovulation in the rabbit[1]. Studies on steroidal control of ovulation in the human lagged partly because for some time progesterone was the only progestational agent available and its effectiveness when taken orally was negligible[2]. Ethisterone, an orally potent progestagen related to 17β-ethinyl testosterone, only became available for clinical use in 1944.

Kurzrok drew attention in 1937 to the fact that during treatment of dysmenorrhoea with oestrone ovulation was inhibited and that this hormone offered a possibility of temporary fertility control[3]. Some years later Albright (1945) suggested that 1 mg of stilboestrol by mouth daily from the first day of the cycle period for the next six weeks would suppress ovulation during this interval; if the patient then wanted to continue the birth control further, she could continue the stilboestrol and take a course of progesterone to cause menstruation[4]. This suggestion went unheeded. The climate for this form of temporary sterilization had not yet appealed to scientists and the gynaecological establishment. The birth control clinic was on the fringe of accepted medical practice. It was not until Dr Abraham Stone and Margaret Sanger invited Gregory Pincus to interest himself in this important aspect of social medicine that an active search for an effective contraceptive regimen began. The pharmaceutical industry had been hard at work synthesizing compounds with progestational activity many times more potent than ethisterone, for it was such an agent that students of reproductive physiology believed could be the key to conception control.

Actually, the seeds for birth control by hormonal methods were sown in March 1919 when Ludwig Haberlandt, Professor of Physiology at Innsbruck, Austria, transplanted ovaries from pregnant rabbits under the skin of fertile adult does and found they became infertile[5]. He foresaw that hormonal sterilization, based on a biological principle, was indeed a possibility. The publication by Wilson and Kurzrok of their observation that dysmenorrhoea occurred mainly in ovulatory women led Sturgis and Albright (1940) to employ injections of oestradiol benzoate every few days during the cycle in an effort to inhibit ovulation and thereby dysmenorrhoea[6,7]. However, ovulation escaped every other month making this regimen only partially effective (Figure 1.1). Greenblatt (1942) used daily stilboestrol suppositories during the cycle in an attempt to overcome dysmenorrhoea by ovulation inhibition with more than moderate success[8]. Lyons (1943) and Haus, Goldzieher and Hamblen (1947) used an oral oestrogen from day 5 to 25 with more or less similar results[9,10]. To offset escape of ovulation when oestrogens alone were employed, Greenblatt (1953, 1954) tried oral oestrogens in

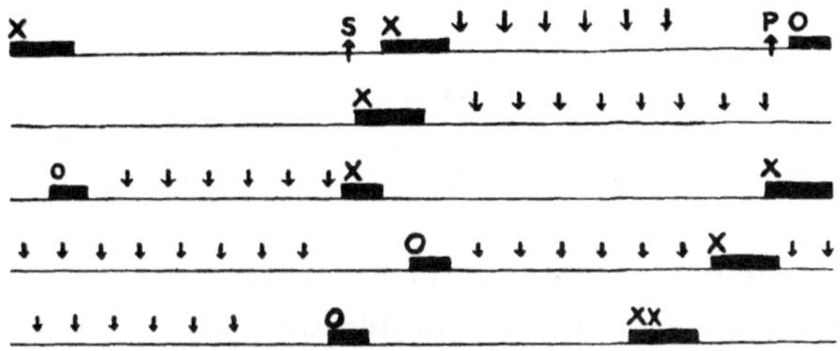

Figure 1.1 Each line represents 2 months. X = cramps; O = no cramps; S = secretory endometrium found by biopsy; P = proliferative endometrium; oblong blocks indicate days of catamenia; arrow indicates day on which 1.7 mg of oestradiol benzoate was administered. It should be noted that on the second and fourth lines there were intervals of 14 days and 13 days respectively between two consecutive courses, which allowed maturation of a follicle to occur and resulted in cramps. However, a third consecutive course started at the end of the fourth line resulted in suppression of ovulation just as a first course would and for the same reason. At onset of cramps with the last period recorded on the fifth line, the patient was given 2 mg of progesterone with no relief whatsoever (XX). (Reproduced by courtesy of *Endocrinology* (1940), **26**, 68)

a continuous manner and in descending doses with the interposition of several days of an oral progestagen to induce menses. Ovulation was successfully inhibited for one year's time (Figure 1.2)[11a, 11b]. In 1957, Rock, Garcia and Pincus used a potent new

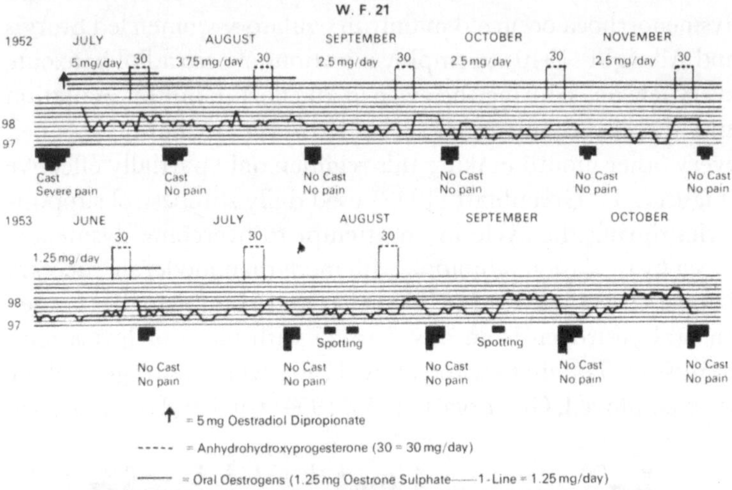

Figure 1.2 Inhibition of ovulation by continuous but descending doses of an oral oestrogen with interposition of short courses of a progestagen. (Reproduced by courtesy of *Am. J. Obstet. Gynecol.* (1954), **68**, 835)

oral progestagen, norethynodrel 30 mg/day, from day 5 to 25 of the cycle in the management of infertility and found that they had successfully inhibited ovulation without much untoward effect or disturbance of the cycle[12].

Table 1.1 Reduction of oestrogen dosage in the combination pill

	Norethynodrel	*EE3ME**
Enovid (Searle)	9.58 mg	150 μg
Enovid E (Searle)	2.5 mg	100 μg

* EE3ME = mestranol

These studies led to the approval in 1959 of the first oral contraceptive pill and a new era in hormonal control of conception burst upon the world (Table 1.1). However, it was not too long before the early enthusiasm for this modality began to fade. The continuous suppression of ovulation over the years led many women to experience disturbing psychogenic and metabolic changes.

A RETROSPECTIVE VIEW OF ORAL CONTRACEPTIVES

An accepted premise in the practice of medicine is that there are virtually no effective medicinal agents that are without possible untoward effects. Unfortunately, the Pill in recent years has been the subject of disturbing reports and has come under considerable scrutiny concerning possible hazards and deleterious effects. Many women, and not a few physicians, are having second thoughts. In view of the publicized warnings, it is well that investigators in the field of reproductive physiology and the pharmaceutical industry are attempting to reduce the risks of the Pill through modification of the progestagen which is to be used in combination with the lowest effective oestrogen dose.

Many side-effects have been attributed to the Pill. Some are trivial, others quite dangerous. Nausea, vomiting, breast engorgement, breakthrough bleeding, weight gain, headaches, chloasma, visual disturbances, and loss of libido are side-effects which may cause some women to abandon the Pill. The most serious condition for which an association with the Pill has been established is thromboembolic disease through an increased tendency to blood clotting[13,14]. The incidence of this disorder appears to be several times higher among women taking oral contraceptives who smoke than among Pill users who do not[15]. The excess mortality from pulmonary embolism or infarction attributed to the use of oral contraceptives was estimated by a group of British investigators to be three deaths per year per

100 000 users. When this figure is weighed against the known risk to maternal life resulting from legal and particularly illegal abortion, along with unknown numbers of suicides which may occur because of unwanted pregnancy, the relative safety of the Pill takes on greater significance (Table 1.2)[16].

Table 1.2 Mortality associated with pregnancy and childbirth, legal abortion, oral contraceptives (by smoking status), and IUDs, by age

Age (years)	*Pregnancy and childbirth**	*Legal abortion†*	*Oral contraceptives‡§*		*IUDs‡*
			Non-smokers	*Smokers*	
15–19	11.1	1.2	1.2	1.4	0.8
20–24	10.0	1.2	1.2	1.4	0.8
25–29	12.5	1.4	1.2	1.4	1.0
30–34	24.9	1.4	1.8	10.4	1.0
35–39	44.0	1.8	3.9	12.8	1.4
40–44	71.4	1.8	6.6	58.4	1.4

* Per 100 000 live birth (excluding abortion), USA, 1972–1974
† Per 100 000 first trimester abortions, USA, 1972–1974
‡ Per 100 000 users per year
§ Estimates by Dr Anrudh K. Jain

Nonetheless, it would be imprudent to ignore the data offered by the Royal College of General Practitioners study (1977), which shows that the incidence of acute myocardial infarction is more than three times greater in oral contraceptive users than in controls, and which also shows a similarly alarming incidence of cerebrovascular accidents (subarachnoid haemorrhage, cerebral haemorrhage, and thrombosis) (Tables 1.2 and 1.3)[17]. However, the impact of the data is defused when one goes on to read that Pill users have a three times greater risk of committing suicide or being murdered than non-users (Table 1.4).

Prolonged use of the Pill has led to aberrations in carbohydrate metabolism, liver function, blood pressure and lipid levels. These changes are temporary, reverting to normal on discontinuation of the Pill. There is an incidence of secondary amenorrhoea, sometimes complicated by persistent lactation, which occurs on discontinuation of the Pill. Fortunately, the resultant infertility may be overcome by clomid with or without hCG or bromergocryptine[18].

Table 1.3 Clinical history of nine women users of oral contraceptives who died from cardiovascular disease

Clinical history	*N*	*Cigarettes smoked/day*	*Age*
Heart disease	3	12; 0; 5	45; 37; 32
Mitral valve disease			
Bundle branch block, age 27			
Fallot's tetralogy			
Toxaemia	3	20; 20; 20	37; 36; 28
None	3	17; 15; 0	37; 36; 35

(After Vessey *et al.*[14])

Table 1.4 Mortality rate of oral contraceptive users per 100000 woman-years

Cause of death	*Ever-users*	*Controls*
Breast cancer	3	6
Acute myocardial infarction	7	2
Cerebrovascular diseases	10	3
Complications of pregnancy	0	2
Suicide–homicide	7	2
Other causes	29	30
Total	56 (58%)	45 (40.9%)

(Modified from Royal College of General Practitioners, 1977, Table II)

The statement that no effective drug can be absolutely safe is understandable and acceptable, but such agents are generally used for the cure of the sick, while the Pill is being administered to normal, healthy women. There are those who hold that any reaction which results in a lengthy illness or death makes the Pill too hazardous and its use unjustifiable. But before reaching such a conclusion, let us examine the consequences to the individual health and national welfare of so-called harmless contraceptive measures, or no contraception at all.

Effective contraceptive methods prevent the 'illness' that is pregnancy. This physiological event may be attended by many side-effects, ranging from nausea to eclampsia and death. For every one million women pregnant between the ages of 20 and 34, there will be 228 who will die as a result of their pregnancy; and for every million women pregnant between the ages of 35 and 44, 576 will die as a result of the pregnancy (Table 1.5). In

Table 1.5 Risk of death from sexual exposure

Method of protection	*Pregnancies*	*Deaths due to pregnancy*	*Deaths due to method*	*Total*
None	880 000	200	0	200
IUD	30 000	7	2	9
Oral contraception	5 000	1	13	14
Diaphragm	120 000	27	0	27
Tubal ligations	17 600	3	150	153
Vaginal hysterectomy	0	0	90	90

1 000 000 women, age 20–34 years, for 1 year

view of these statistics, which were published in 1968 by the International Planned Parenthood Federation, one may ask, 'Is pregnancy safe?' Consider the fact that for every million women who practice rhythm for birth control, about 240 000 will conceive, and about half as many will become pregnant who use the diaphragm and/or spermicidal jellies. How many of these women will die as a result of their pregnancy?

Admittedly, there is reason for concern for users of the Pill because of the fear of thromboembolic disease, the possibility of cerebrovascular accidents, and the spectre of cancer. As to the first, there appears to be a legitimate basis for concern, and any woman with a history of phlebitis or varicosities should not be placed on the Pill (Table 1.6). Should signs of phlebitis develop, the Pill should be discontinued and precautionary measures taken until the condition subsides. As to cerebrovascular accidents, a cause and effect relationship has not been established,

Table 1.6 Contraindications for oral contraceptives

Smoking	History of:
Hypertension	Thrombosis
Diabetes	Heart disease
Hyperlipidaemia	Toxaemia of pregnancy
Obesity	Abnormal uterine bleeding
Acquired headaches	Impaired liver function

but women who develop headaches or visual disturbances on the Pill should go on to some other contraceptive method. As to cancer, there is no evidence to support the assumption that the Pill will cause cancer. Indeed, clinicians with the greatest experience in the field of oral contraception feel that there may be a decrease in the incidence of cervical, endometrial and breast cancer. This writer earnestly believes this to be the case. After more than two decades of extensive use of the Pill, he has not encountered a single case of endometrial or mammary cancer attributed to the drug, notwithstanding the report of Silverberg and Makowski[19]. The Advisory Committee of Obstetrics and Gynecology to the Food and Drug Administration, after study of adverse reactions, concluded that 'no effective drug can be absolutely safe'. When potential hazards and the value of the Pill were balanced, the Committee found the 'ratio of benefit to risk sufficiently high to justify the designation safe . . .'.

The Royal College of General Practitioners in Britain completed a massive study that should lay to rest recurring fears of serious side-effects. More than 15000 users of oral contraceptives, plus a control group of roughly equal size, were examined periodically and every illness or complaint of each woman was recorded for a period of 4 years. They reported that 'not a single previously unsuspected important adverse effect of the Pill has been revealed by the study so far, and several suspected risks have been shown to be small or non-existent'. A serious adverse effect appears to be hypertension, which may increase with use and age up to about 5% of Pill-takers. Another untoward effect of the Pill is the occasional case of hepatoma. One specific fear discovered to be unfounded was that the Pill increased the incidence of diabetes. Moreover, the side-effects beneficial to health were not inconsequential; for example, a lower rate of benign breast tumours and protection against ovarian cysts and iron-deficiency anaemia. The latter finding is of particular importance for women in developing countries.

The occurrence of thrombophlebitis in a former president of the United States has focused attention on the natural history of this disease. It is a far more frequent cause of death than hitherto suspected. Although oral contraceptives increase the incidence of thromboembolic phenomena, the weighted incidence is less than what was first suspected.

IMPROVED FORMULATIONS OF ORAL CONTRACEPTIVES

The Pill was approved for contraceptive use in November 1959. It contained norethynodrel 9.85 mg and mestranol 0.15 mg and was known as Enovid®. Its development has undoubtedly been the single most important event in the control of human fertility in the 20th century. In May 1962 a pill containing 10 mg of norethindrone and 0.6 mg of mestranol became available; it was known as Ortho-Novum 10®. Whereas the progestagen in Enovid was slightly oestrogenic and devoid of androgenic effects, the progestagen in Ortho-Novum 10 was not oestrogenic but slightly androgenic. Other progestagens are anti-oestrogenic while some have highly potent progestational activity. Therefore, not all progestagens are alike or elicit similar metabolic reactions. Furthermore, they vary greatly in potency when measured by the delay of menses test. Whereas norgestrel

Table 1.7 Relation of structure to potency of oestrane derivatives

Structure	*Differences from nor-testosterone*			*Delay of menses test*
	17β-substituent	*Acetate*	*Other changes*	
Norethindrone 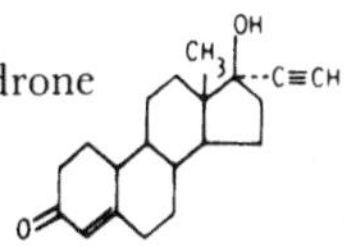	Ethinyl	—	—	15 mg
Norethynodrel 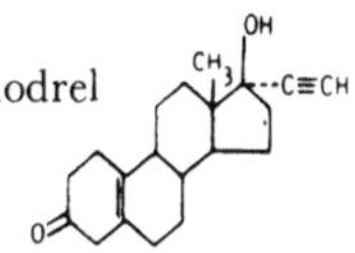	Ethinyl	—	$\Delta^{5(10)}$ instead of Δ^4	13.8 mg
Norethindrone acetate 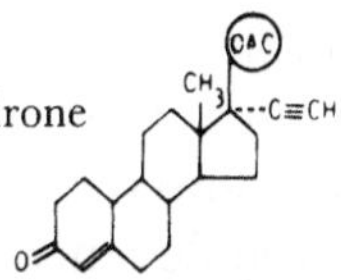	Ethinyl	17	—	7.5 mg
Ethynodiol diacetate 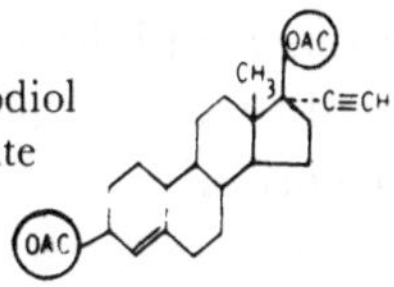	Ethinyl	3β, 17	—	1 mg
Norgestrel 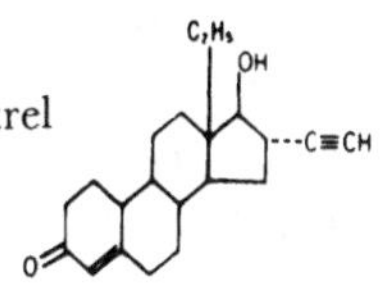	Ethinyl	—	C_2H_5 in 18th position	0.5 mg

requires only 0.5 mg for a positive test, it requires 10–15 mg of norethindrone (Table 1.7)[20a, 20b].

In 1969, reports of thromboembolic disease and myocardial infarction were said to correlate with the oestrogen content[21, 22]. In rapid succession a large number of progestagens, some with distinctive properties in combination with either mestranol or ethinyloestradiol in various combinations and in decreasing dosages, were in manufacture so that over two dozen preparations of combination and sequential pills for contraception became available throughout the world (Table 1.8).

Table 1.8

Product	*Oestrogen*	*Progestagen*
Enovid 10	150 μg EE3ME*	9.85 mg Norethynodrel
Orthonovum	60 μg EE3ME*	10.00 mg Norethindrone
Orthonovum 1/50	50 μg EE3ME*	1.00 mg Norethindrone
Lo estrin	30 μg EE†	1.50 mg Norethindrone acetate
Lo ovral	30 μg EE	0.30 mg Norgestrel

*EE3ME = Mestranol
†EE = Ethinyloestradiol

The reduction in the oestrogen and progestagen content of the Pill did not appreciably compromise contraceptive potential, while untoward effects were considerably lowered. However, breakthrough bleeding became quite troublesome. Then in 1977 the Royal College of General Practitioners published their findings that a correlation existed between the magnitude of the progestagen and the incidence of hypertension[23]. Conflicting reports have appeared on the effect of synthetic oestrogens and of various progestagens on high density lipoproteins (HDL). *Efforts are now being directed at a Pill which minimizes metabolic change, decreases the incidence of breakthrough bleeding or spotting, without compromising efficacy. It is with these goals in mind that a triphasic Pill has been developed in the belief that many of the undesirable side-effects can be circumvented while maintaining almost 100% conception control.*

CONCLUSIONS

Conjugal life should not be hampered by fear of conception. The Pill has served to unfetter women from the agonies of an unwanted pregnancy, and has thus done much to improve the psyche and well-being of many. The limitation of family size to the number of children who are desired and who can be cared for by the parents is good for the family unit and for society. Every child should be wanted and planned for, with a design for his future welfare. Closely allied to this theme of birth control for the family unit is the greater and weightier problem of national and international concern – the population explosion. High density populations foster social stress, poverty, hostility, violence and moral degradation. Even laboratory rats – packed too many in one cage – become socially maladjusted and soon devour one another. The ultimate goal of the Pill is safety and efficacy, and to provide a means whereby the destiny of man and the welfare of our world will not be left to chance or to sexual desire alone.

References

1. Makepeace, A. W., Weinstein, G. L. and Friedman, M. H. (1937). The effect of progestin and progesterone on ovulation in the rabbit. *Am. J. Physiol.*, **119**, 512
2. Greenblatt, R. B. (1952). Progesterone. In *Office Endocrinology*, p. 373 (Springfield, III: Charles C. Thomas)
3. Kurzrok, R. (1937). The prospects for hormonal sterilization. *J. Contracept.*, **2**, 27
4. Albright, F. (1945). Disorders of the female gonads. In J. H. Musser (ed.), *Internal Medicine – its Theory and Practice* (Philadelphia: Lea and Febiger). Quoted in Editorial, *Hum. Fert.*, **10**, 80 (1945)
5. Haberlandt, L. (1921). Ueber hormonale Sterilisierung des wiblichen Tierkörpers. *Münch. Med. Wochenschr.*, **68**, 1577
6. Wilson, L. and Kruzrok, R. (1940). Uterine contractility in functional dysmenorrhea. *Endocrinology*, **27**, 23
7. Sturgis, S. H. and Albright, F. (1940). Mechanism of estrin therapy in the relief of dysmenorrhea. *Endocrinology*, **26**, 68

8. Greenblatt, R. B. (1942). Diethylstilbestrol suppository medication in dysmenorrhea. *J. South Carolina Med. Assoc.*, **38**, 3
9. Lyon, R. A. (1943). Relief of essential dysmenorrhea with ethinyl estradiol. *Surg. Gynecol. Obstet*, **77**, 657
10. Haus, L., Goldzieher, J. W. and Hamblen, E. C. (1947). Dysmenorrhea and ovulation. Correlation of the effect of estrogen therapy on pain, the endometrium, and basal body temperature. *Am. J. Obstet. Gynecol.*, **54**, 820
11a. Greenblatt, R. B. (1952). Dysmenorrhea. In *Office Endocrinology*, p. 203 (Springfield, III: Charles C. Thomas)
11b. Greenblatt, R. B., Hammond, D. O. and Clark, S. L. (1954). Membranous dysmenorrhea: Studies in etiology and treatment. *Am. J. Obstet. Gynecol.*, **68**, 835
12. Rock, J., Garcia, C. R. and Pincus, G. (1957). Synthetic progestins in the normal human menstrual cycle. *Recent Progr. Horm. Res.*, **13**, 323
13. Royal College of General Practitioners (1967). Oral contraception and thromboembolic disease
14. Vessey, M. P., McPherson, K. and Johnson, B. (1977). Mortality among women participating in the Oxford/Family Planning Association contraceptive study. *Lancet*, **2**, 731
15. Jain, A. K. (1976). Cigarette smoking, use of oral contraceptives and myocardial infarction. *Am. J. Obstet. Gynecol.*, **126**, 301
16. Tietze, C. and Lewit, S. (1977). Mortality and fertility control. *Int. J. Gynaecol. Obstet.*, **15**, 100
17. Greenblatt, R. B., Nezhat, C. and McNamara, V. P. (1979). Appropriate contraception for middle-aged women. *J. Biosoc. Sci.*(Suppl. 6), 119
18. Greenblatt, R. B. (ed.) (1979). *Induction of Ovulation.* (Philadelphia: Lea and Febiger)
19. Silverberg, S. G. and Makowski, E. L. (1975). Endometrial carcinoma in young women taking oral contraceptives. *Obstet. Gynecol.*, **46**, 503
20a. Greenblatt, R. B., Clark, S. L. and Jungck, E. C. (1958). A new test for efficacy of progestational agents. *Ann. N.Y. Acad. Sci.*, **71**, 717
20b. Swyer, G. I. M. and Little, V. (1962). Actions and uses of orally active progestational steroids. *Proc. R. Soc. Med.*, **55**, 861
21. Vessey, M. P. and Doll, R. (1969). Investigation of relationship between use of oral contraceptives and thromboembolic disease. A further report. *Br. Med. J.*, **2**, 651
22. Sartwell, P. E., Masi, A. T., Arthes, F. G., Greene, G. R. and Smith, H. E. (1969). Thromboembolism and oral contraceptives: an epidemiologic case-control study. *Am. J. Epidemiol.*, **90**, 365
23. Royal College of General Practitioners (1977). Effect of hypertension and benign breast disease of progestogen component in combined oral contraceptives. *Lancet*, **2**, 624

2
The rationale for a new triphasic contraceptive

U. LACHNIT-FIXSON

Since the introduction of the Pill, more than 20 years ago, research in this field has been directed towards improving the tolerance and cycle control of these preparations and – even more important – towards reducing their influence on certain parameters of the haemostatic system and metabolic functions, thus increasing their safety from the medical point of view. These improvements have been achieved by reducing the dose of both components, introducing new and more effective progestagens, and by changing the oestrogen:progestagen ratio in the various preparations.

In my own opinion, a well balanced oestrogen:progestagen ratio is of paramount importance, especially when one takes into account that certain progestagens can counteract several unwanted metabolic effects of oestrogens and vice versa[1,2]. Furthermore one has to consider that a fixed dose regimen imposes a very unnatural situation on a woman.

During the normal menstrual cycle there are the well-known characteristic fluctuations in the plasma levels of β-oestradiol and progesterone (Figure 2.1)[3]. Mimicking them as closely as possible should further improve tolerance and cycle control of oral contraceptives, even when using relatively low total quantities of both steroids.

For quite a long time the oestrogen was regarded, so to speak, as the 'root of all evil' in hormonal contraception[4–7] and reduction of the daily oestrogen dose was considered to be the ultimate goal.

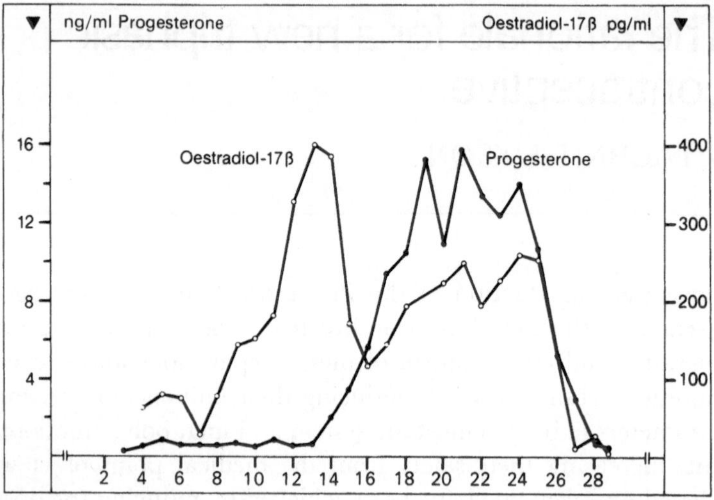

Figure 2.1 Plasma levels of 17β-oestradiol and progesterone during the course of the normal menstrual cycle

However, in the last few years a series of studies has been published that throws an interesting light on the role of progestagen, especially concerning blood pressure changes and disturbances of lipid and carbohydrate metabolism[2,8–12,18], so that an acceptable reduction of the progestagen component should be of great importance as well. One may summarize all recent findings in a recommendation given by the WHO in 1978: it is advisable to use the lowest possible effective and acceptable dose of steroid contraceptive preparations so as to minimize any potential risk[13]. Coming back to my favourite idea, let me add: preferably preparations adapted to the phases of the normal menstrual cycle.

Our first step in this direction was the development of a biphasic preparation with an 11/10 regimen. It has the following composition:

11 coated tablets of 0.05 mg ethinyloestradiol + 0.5 mg levonorgestrel
10 coated tablets of 0.05 mg ethinyloestradiol + 0.125 mg levonorgestrel

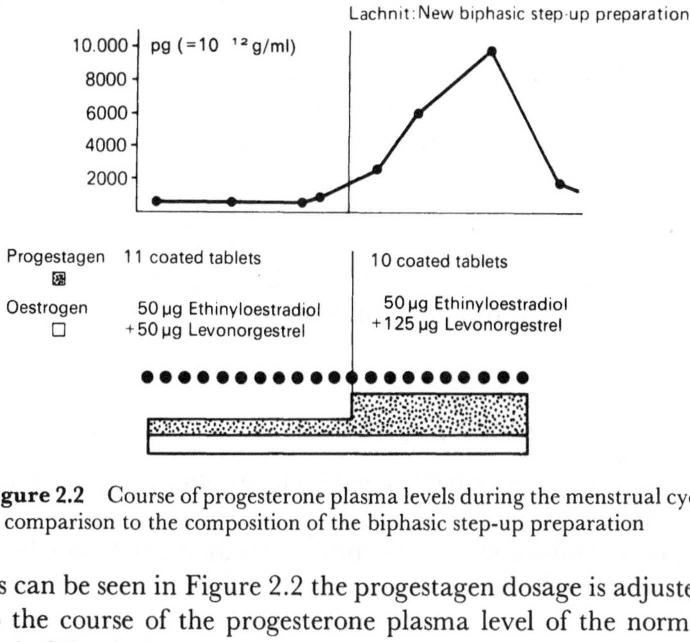

Figure 2.2 Course of progesterone plasma levels during the menstrual cycle in comparison to the composition of the biphasic step-up preparation

As can be seen in Figure 2.2 the progestagen dosage is adjusted to the course of the progesterone plasma level of the normal cycle. We tried to create a 'luteal phase' very similar in length to that of the normal menstrual cycle.

This type of preparation was introduced 1974 in Germany and subsequently in several other countries. Especially in Central European countries it gained wide acceptance, because of good cycle control and tolerance. Another interesting aspect: weight problems are almost non-existent with the step-up regimen. The total amount of progestagen administered per cycle is extremely low and yet the daily dose of oestrogen is only 0.05 mg. Step-up preparations provide an equally high contraceptive security as classical combination products, and, in this respect, there is a definite advantage over the earlier sequential preparations which failed to obtain a comparable reliability despite a much higher oestrogen dosage[14,15].

Bearing in mind the varying oestrogen plasma levels, it then seemed logical in 1973 to attempt the development of a step-up preparation containing the lowest possible quantity of *both hormone components*. In doing so, 3-phase-structured models were chosen that would provide increased oestrogen doses for 5 days in mid-cycle, thus fitting in with the normal pre-ovulatory oestrogen peak. Just as in the normal cycle we subdivided the follicular phase into a post-menstrual phase of 6 days duration and a peri-ovulatory one of 5 days duration, whereas we kept the 10-day luteal phase which has proved so successfully in the biphasic regimen. Here you can see the composition of the two preparations which were to undergo extensive clinical investigation.

Preparation 1: SH B 264 AB

6 coated tablets of 0.03 mg ethinyloestradiol + 0.05 mg levonorgestrel
5 coated tablets of 0.04 mg ethinyloestradiol + 0.075 mg levonorgestrel
10 coated tablets of 0.03 mg ethinyloestradiol + 0.125 mg levonorgestrel

Preparation 2: SH B 261 AB

6 coated tablets of 0.03 mg ethinyloestradiol + 0.05 mg levonorgestrel
5 coated tablets of 0.05 mg ethinyloestradiol + 0.05 mg levonorgestrel

10 coated tablets of 0.04 mg ethinyloestradiol + 0.125 mg levonorgestrel

Even in the first pilot studies, conducted to ascertain the mode of action of such models, it was shown that such an arrangement – compared to other low-dose preparations – resulted in clearly improved cycle control[16,17].

I shall report on the extended clinical trials later on, in the third part of our conference. Just to anticipate the result of the comparative trial between the two versions: the final choice fell on the trial preparation SH B 264 AB.

In conclusion it is to be demonstrated here how well the hormone content in the different phases of the SH B 264 AB-medication cycle is adjusted to the plasma levels of β-oestradiol and progesterone in the corresponding phases of the normal menstrual cycle (Figures 2.3 and 2.4).

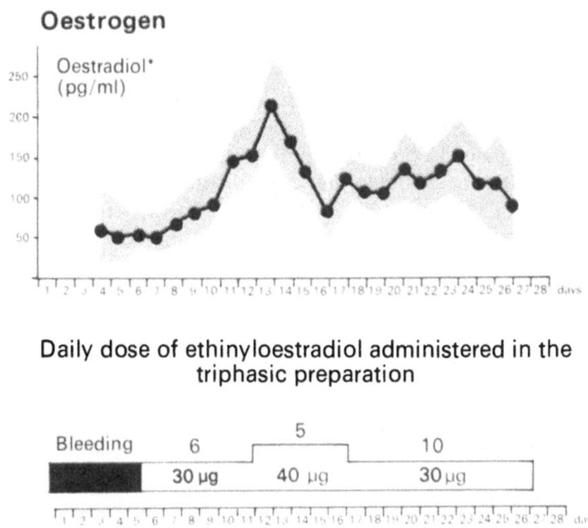

Figure 2.3 Adjustment of oestrogen dosage in the triphasic preparation to the different phases of the menstrual cycle. This applies from the second cycle onwards as treatment begins on the first day of bleeding in the first cycle. * Normal oestradiol values in the serum during the ovulatory cycle (mean value + standard deviation) (Acc. to Schmidt-Matthiesen)

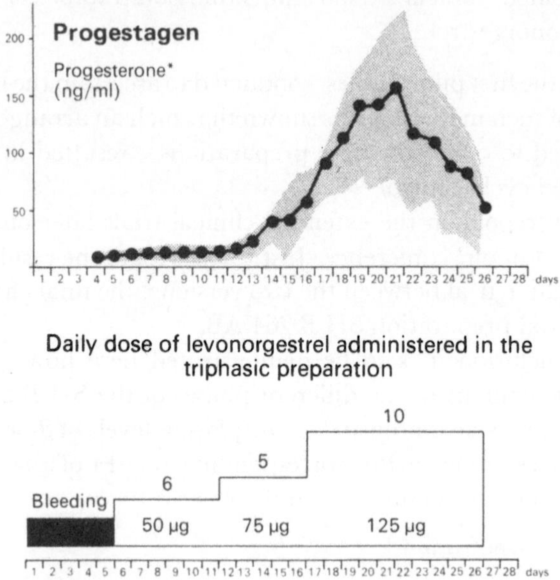

Figure 2.4 Adjustment of progestagen dosage in the triphasic preparation to the different phases of the menstrual cycle. This applies from the second cycle onwards as treatment begins on the first day of bleeding in the first cycle. * Normal progesterone values in the serum during the ovulatory cycle (mean value + standard deviation) (Acc. to Schmidt-Matthiesen)

References

1. Briggs, M. H. (1975). Effects of oral progestogens on estrogen-induced changes in plasma proteins. *J. Reprod. Med.*, **15**, 3, 100
2. Briggs, M. H. (1978). Biochemical basis for evaluating oral contraceptives. Int. Symp. *A Reappraisal of Fertility Control, Benefits vs Risks*, Montreal, Canada
3. Nocke, W., Leyendecker, G. (1972). Neue Erkenntnisse über die endokrine Physiologie des menstruellen Cyclus. *Gynäkologe*, **5**, 39
4. Combined Oral Contraceptives (1970). A Statement by the Committee on Safety of Drugs. *Br. Med. J.*, **2**, 231
5. Inman, W. H. W. *et al.* (1970). Thromboembolic disease and the steroidal content of oral contraceptives. A Report to the Committee on Safety of Drugs. *Br. Med. J.*, **2**, 203

6. Oestrogens and Thromboembolism (1970). *Br. Med. J.*, **2**, 189
7. Royal College of General Practitioners (1974). *Oral Contraceptives and Health*. (London: Pitman)
8. Arntzenius, A. C. *et al.* (1978). Reduced high-density lipoprotein in women aged 40–41 using oral contraceptives. *Lancet*, **8076**, 1221
9. Bradley, D. D. *et al.*(1978). Serum high density-lipoprotein cholesterol in women using oral contraceptives, estrogen and progestins. *N. Engl. J. Med.*, **299**, 17
10. Larsson-Cohn, U., Wallentin, L. and Zador, G. (1979). Plasma lipids and high density lipoproteins during oral contraception with different combinations of ethinyl estradiol and levonorgestrel. *Horm. Metab. Res.*, **11**, 437
11. Rössner, S. (1978). Lowering of HDL cholesterol by oral contraceptives. *Lancet*, **2**, 269
12. Wynn, V. *et al.*(1979). Comparison of effects of different combined oral-contraceptive formulations on carbohydrate and lipid metabolism. *Lancet*, 1045
13. Steroid contraception and the risk of neoplasia (1978). WHO-Technical Report 619
14. Lachnit, U. (1974). Bericht über die erweiterte klinische prüfung eines neuen Zwei-Stufen-Präparates. *Ther. D. Gegenw.*, **113**, 1486
15. Lachnit, U. (1975). Einführung und weitere Ergebnisse zur klinischen Prüfung von Sequilar. *Med. Mitt. Schering*, **5**, 2
16. Schneider, W. H. F., Lachnit-Fixson, U., Schmid, R. and Spona, J. (1977). Zur kontrazeptiven Wirksamkeit von Dreistufenpräparaten. *Med. Klin.*, **72**, 2081
17. Schneider, W. H. F., Spona, J., Schmid, R. and Lachnit-Fixson, U. (1977). Efficacy of three-phase oral contraceptives. Int. Symp. on Hormonal Contraception, Utrecht, Netherlands (Amsterdam: Excerpta Medica)
18. Royal College of General Practitioners (1977). Effect on hypertension and benign breast disease of progestagen component in combined oral contraceptives. *Lancet*, **2**, 624

3
The normal menstrual cycle and oral contraceptives: the physiological basis for a triphasic approach

G. VIRGINIA UPTON

INTRODUCTION

The development of the oral contraceptive (OC) represents one of the most significant scientific achievements of this century. This significance is attributed principally to the fact that its practical application has had such a powerful impact on all aspects of society with far-reaching consequences.

The aim of oral contraception was, and still is, the blockade of ovulation. It was known as far back as the 1940s that oestrogens (E) could inhibit ovulation in humans during successive treatment cycles but this blockade was temporary and unpredictable. Ovulation that did occur despite oestrogen ingestion was referred to as an 'escape phenomenon'.

As early as 1897 Beard postulated that progesterone (P) inhibited ovulation during pregnancy[1]. Subsequent studies established the fact that progesterone did inhibit ovulation in the rabbit[2] and in the rat[3]. These observations were also confirmed in humans. Investigators looking for a practical OC reasoned that since the oestrogen blockade was unreliable, a progestational that was orally active and could inhibit ovulation would provide a reasonable alternative approach. The search for such a progestational was pursued vigorously. The goal was to find an agent that would prevent ovulation by inhibiting secretion of pituitary gonadotropins and yet produce a reversible antifertility effect when the drug was withdrawn.

Subsequently, it was demonstrated that norethynodrel depressed the secretion of pituitary gonadotropins. In 1956 Rock[4] first established that ovulation was inhibited in humans by norethynodrel but the frequency of spotting and bleeding encountered was high. Rock suggested that oestrogen be added to the regimen to help in maintaining the endometrium; thus mestranol was introduced as the oestrogenic component. In 1960, Enovid®, (9.85 mg norethynodrel plus 0.150 mg mestranol), became the first oral contraceptive approved by the FDA. Widespread clinical trials conducted by Dr Edris Rice-Wray in Puerto Rico demonstrated excellent contraceptive efficacy with this preparation[5].

This demonstration was a milestone in history and led to the widespread use of oral contraception as a socially acceptable method of family planning[6]. Many oral contraceptives were subsequently developed and marketed. Unfortunately, the doses of steroid contained in these early formulations were very high and the side-effects that appeared made it imperative that new formulations be produced. Of necessity, a variety of OCs with altered oestrogen:progestagen ratios followed, each product claiming superiority over the others.

STRATEGIES

Addressing the problem of side-effects, the strategies have been as follows:

(1) Reduction of steroid dosage,
(2) Development of new steroids,
(3) Introduction of new modes of administration.

Reduction of steroid dosage

Both oestrogen and progestagen dosages have been progressively reduced over the years resulting in many different formulations and ratios.

Since the more serious adverse side-effects had implicated oestrogen as the culprit, the aim has been first to reduce the oestrogen. Because the ratio of oestrogen to progestagen is a major consideration[7], the reduction in progestagen followed. Recognition of the synergistic effect of progestagens with ethinyl oestrogens permitted marked reductions in total steroid content. Small amounts of ethinyl oestrogens combined with small

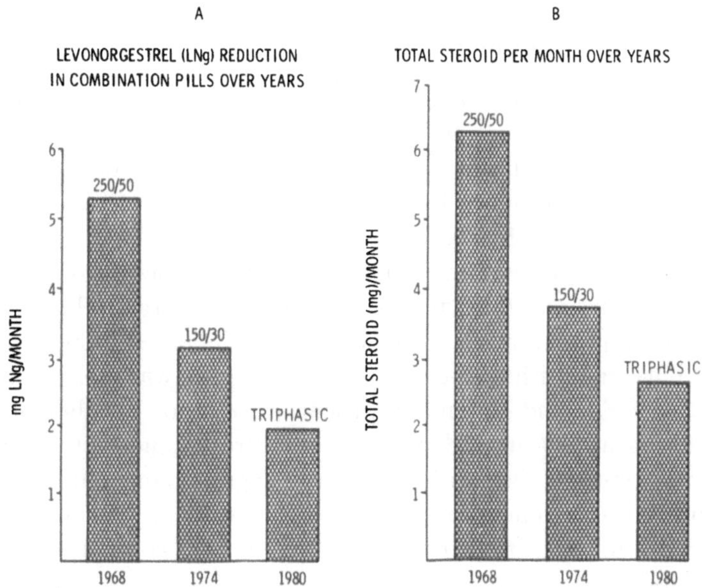

Figure 3.1 Panel A: The total levonorgestrel (mg) per month in three different OCs depicting the reduction over the years as shown. Products represented are: 250 μg LNg + 50 μg EE, 150 μg LNg + 30 μg EE; the new triphasic preparation. Panel B: The total EE + LNg content (mg) per month in the three OCs as shown in Panel A depicting the reduction over the years as shown

amounts of progestagen have as much antiovulatory activity as much larger amounts of ethinyl oestrogen alone[8].

As an example, three norgestrel products are shown in Figure 3.1. The total monthly dose of norgestrel has been consistently reduced over the years culminating in the new 'ultra' low triphasic formulation, which shows about a 40% reduction in this hormone (panel A). In the same figure (Panel B) the total monthly dose of combined steroid reflects the reduction in the oestrogenic component as well. In retrospect, a total monthly dose of 2.6 mg for the new triphasic preparation, compared to the original 210 mg for Enovid, represents a reduction of 98.7% in total steroid per month – a remarkable achievement!

Development of new steroids

The search for new steroids culminated in the use of ethinyloestradiol (EE) or mestranol in most of the pills. Since mestranol must be metabolized first to EE in order to be biologically active, and since much less EE is required to prevent ovulation, ethinyloestradiol has been used preferentially.

Of all the progestational steroids developed the most significant advance was the synthesis of norgestrel. Norgestrel proved to be a potent progestational without inherent oestrogenic activity and with anti-oestrogenic activity. It was biologically active *per se* and had many properties superior to other progestationals. Quite independent of oestrogen, norgestrel had contraceptive effects within the entire hypothalamic–pituitary–gonadal axis. These properties coupled with its potency permitted marked reductions in total steroid content of the combination pill.

Introduction of new modes of administration

Figure 3.2 schematically compares the timing of the administration of oestrogen and progestagen in different OCs with the endogenous hormone levels found during the normal menstrual cycle. The original combination pill, the sequential pill, the biphasic approach and, finally, the triphasic approach are shown. It is important to note that the original sequential pill utilized unopposed oestrogen for 16 days and progestagen combined with an oestrogen for only 5 days. The newer biphasic approach differs markedly from the sequential because unopposed oestrogen is never encountered during the cycle. Similarly, the triphasic pill is always an EE/levonorgestrel

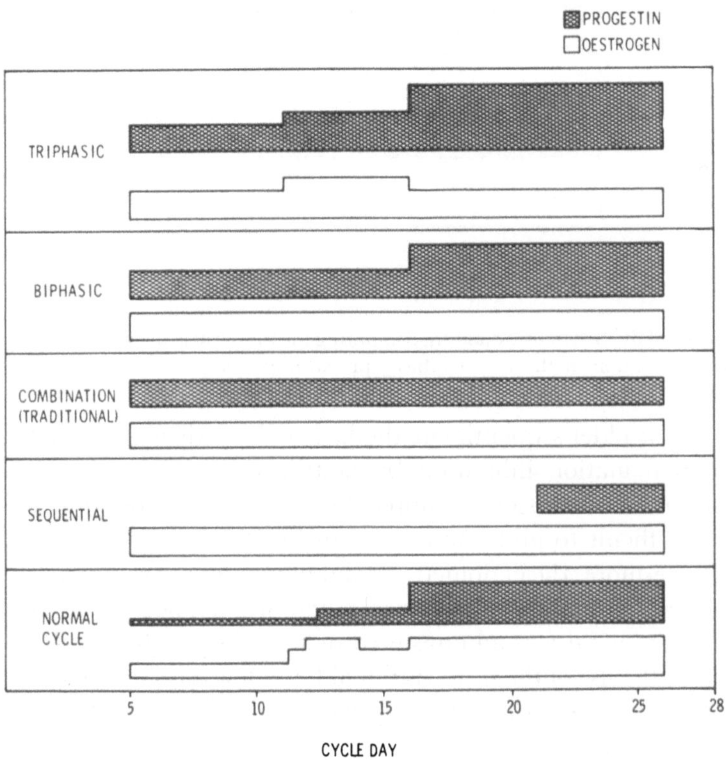

Figure 3.2 Schematic diagram showing the timing of administration of the individual components (oestrogen and progestagen) of various contraceptives compared to the endogenous steroid changes during a normal menstrual cycle

(LNg) combination throughout the 21 days of administration. In addition, an attempt is made with the triphasic regimen to mimic the naturally-occurring rise and fall of E and P by varying the doses of EE and LNg (see Figure 3.3).

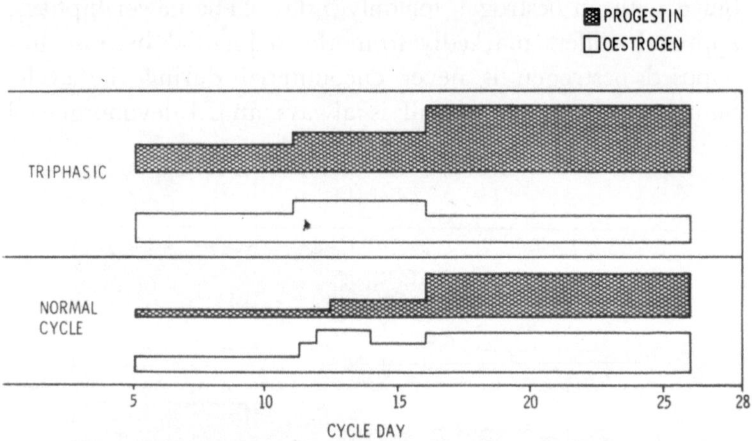

Figure 3.3 Schematic diagram comparing the timing of exogenous hormone administration of the new triphasic preparation compared to endogenous hormone changes during a normal menstrual cycle

In the older sequential method, total dependence was placed upon ovulation inhibition by oestrogen. Since it had been known that oestrogen was unreliable as an inhibitor of ovulation, it is difficult to understand why this method was used at all. Furthermore, the endometrium did not undergo profound progestational changes and cervical mucus was unaffected since the progestational was administered only in the late luteal phase. Thus, the use of the progestational for so few days so late in the cycle provided little contraceptive support to the oestrogenic component.

The new triphasic approach introduces the combination steroid in a step-wise fashion as is observed in the normal menstrual cycle (Figure 3.3). Advantage is taken of the well-known physiological events at midcycle and the known synergism of EE and LNg by introducing increased amounts of these steroids before the physiological gonadotropin surge to ensure inhibition of ovulation. The critical peri-ovulatory period is well spanned with dosages of EE and LNg known to inhibit ovulation even when used alone, obviating the problems that had occurred with the older sequentials.

MODE OF ACTION OF THE TRADITIONAL OCs

Before the advent of the enlightened knowledge in neuroendocrinology and the new radioimmunoassay technology, the concept prevailed that inhibition of ovulation was by direct effect on the pituitary gland to inhibit LH and FSH. But with newer techniques it has been shown that the OCs, particularly those with a high oestrogen content, can directly affect the hypothalamus to inhibit luteinizing hormone (gonadotropin) releasing hormone (LHRH; GnRH)[9–13] and can also cause direct suppression of the pituitary gland[9,13–18]. Norgestrel itself, at a high enough dose, can directly produce inhibition at the hypothalamic level[19].

As reliance on oestrogens as ovulation inhibitors decreased, particularly with the new lower dose pills, the importance of the role of the progestational component assumed greater significance.

Because levonorgestrel has contraceptive effects within the entire hypothalamic–gonadal axis independent of the presence of oestrogen, this unique steroid provides a number of additional mechanisms reinforcing contraceptive efficacy.

Among these properties, its ability to suppress hypothalamic LHRH secretion, thus blocking the midcycle gonadotropin surge, and consequently blocking ovulation, is paramount. In addition, the following contraceptive actions of norgestrel have been demonstrated[20–23] (see Figure 3.4).

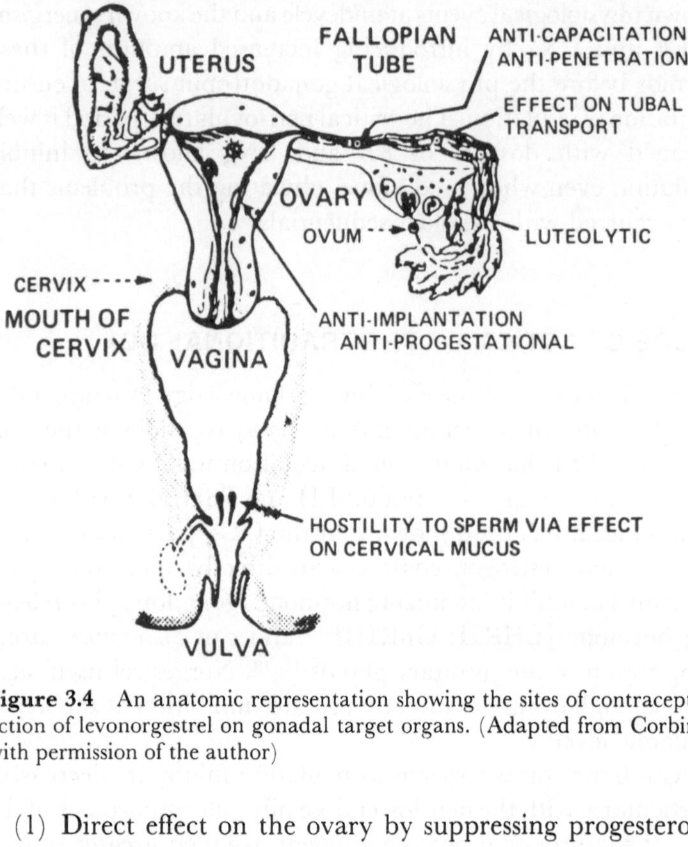

Figure 3.4 An anatomic representation showing the sites of contraceptive action of levonorgestrel on gonadal target organs. (Adapted from Corbin [25] with permission of the author)

(1) Direct effect on the ovary by suppressing progesterone output.

(2) Alteration of cervical mucus with inhibition of sperm transport. The cervical mucus becomes scanty, viscous and cellular and exhibits reduced spinnbarkeit and ferning.

(3) Direct endometrial changes preventing implantation.

It has been demonstrated that reduction in the steroid content of the OCs results in less suppression of the hypothalamic–pituitary–ovarian axis.

Table 3.1 Comparison of hormone levels† in women using mechanical contraception, standard or low-oestrogen oral contraceptives‡

Method	*Number of subjects*	*Oestradiol (pg/ml)*	*Progesterone (ng/nl)*	*Testosterone (ng/ml)*	*FSH (mIU/ml)*	*LH (mIU/ml)*
Mechanical contraception	20	175.9 ± 18.8*	5.0 ± 0.9	34.1 ± 3.6	7.3 ± 1.2	16.1 ± 3.2
Low-dose oestrogen OC						
35 μg oestrogen	10	88.0 ± 38.4	1.9 ± 1.1	30.5 ± 4.2	4.5 ± 0.8	8.0 ± 1.1
Standard OC						
50 μg⁺ oestrogen	17	20.8 ± 2.1	0.3 ± 0.04	24.7 ± 2.1	2.6 ± 0.4	3.9 ± 0.4

* Mean ± SE
† Cycle day 17–21
‡ Adapted from Spellacy *et al.*[9]

In a recent study by Spellacy *et al.*[9], the hypothalamic–pituitary–ovarian axis was evaluated in 47 women who were divided into three groups: 20 women using mechanical contraception (controls), 17 women using oral contraceptives containing 50 μg or more of oestrogen (high oestrogen: HE), and 10 women using oral contraceptives containing 35 μg of oestrogen (low oestrogen: LE).

Between days 17 to 21 of their cycle, basal levels of hormones were measured. Table 3.1 lists the levels of FSH, LH, oestradiol (E), progesterone (P), and testosterone (T) for each group. The HE group showed significant reductions in basal levels of FSH, LH, E, P and T whereas the LE group showed a decrease in only E.

It can readily be seen in Table 3.1 that basal levels of steroid decreased with increasing doses of oestrogen. Although the data would implicate oestrogen as the causal agent, these pills are combinations of oestrogen and progestagen and it must be assumed that both components contribute to the observed effect.

In addition, these 47 women were given consecutive i.v. administrations of 0.5, 5.0 and 50 μg of gonadotropin releasing hormone (GnRH) as a bolus at 90 minute intervals. Plasma levels of FSH and LH were determined every 30 minutes for 4.5 hours.

Figures 3.5 and 3.6 show the FSH and LH levels respectively over time. The high oestrogen group revealed retarded and blunted plasma hormonal (FSH and LH) responses to the graded consecutive i.v. doses of GnRH. In contrast, control subjects responded to the GnRH with significantly earlier and greater elevations in plasma LH and FSH. The low oestrogen group yielded gonadotropin responses to GnRH with levels falling between the responses of the high oestrogen group and control.

It should be noted that all of the OCs used in Spellacy's trial block ovulation. Since delayed and suppressed responses to the

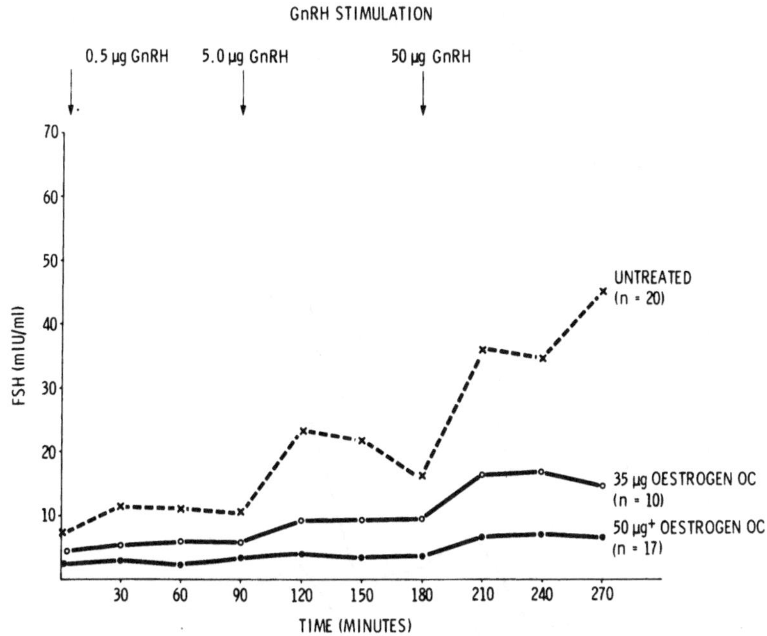

Figure 3.5 Plasma FSH values in three groups of women in response to graded consecutive doses (0.5, 5.0, 50 μg) of GnRH administered i.v. as a bolus at 90-minute intervals. The three groups shown are: 20 women using mechanical contraception (controls); 17 women using oral contraceptives with high oestrogen (50 μg or higher) and 10 women using a low oestrogen (35 μg) oral contraceptive. (Adapted from Spellacy *et al.*[9] with permission of author and publisher)

provocative GnRH stimulus are evident, albeit to varying degrees, the OCs apparently are suppressing both the hypothalamus and the pituitary. The low oestrogen group suppressed the hypothalamic–pituitary axis to a much lesser degree; this suppression is not evidenced by fasting levels of LH, FSH, P and T but rather by lower basal oestradiol levels and by a blunted LH response to 50 μg GnRH.

Since the low oestrogen OCs retain their ability to block ovulation despite the lesser suppression of the hypothalamic–

pituitary axis, it follows that lower oestrogen OCs should be used whenever possible because fewer systemic side-effects and longterm sequelae such as post-pill amenorrhoea may be predicted.

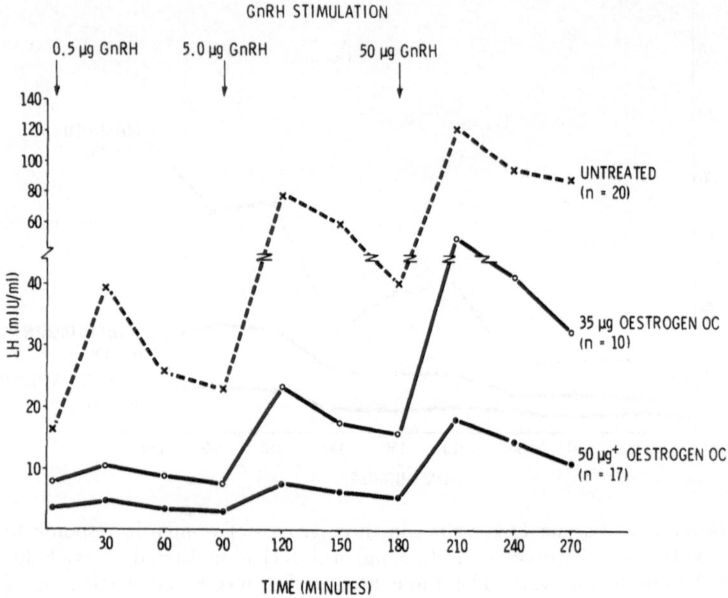

Figure 3.6 Plasma LH values in the same three groups of women as shown in Figure 3.5 under the same experimental conditions. (Adapted from Spellacy *et al.*[9] with permission of author and publisher)

MODE OF ACTION OF THE NEW TRIPHASIC ORAL CONTRACEPTIVE*

The new triphasic composition and delivery is as follows:

6 tablets of 30 µg ethinyloestradiol and 50 µg levonorgestrel
5 tablets of 40 µg ethinyloestradiol and 75 µg levonorgestrel
10 tablets of 30 µg ethinyloestradiol and 125 µg levonorgestrel

*WL-49(50); SH B 264 AB

By analogy to the experiments of Spellacy we can assume that the new triphasic contraceptive, which contains slightly less oestrogen than the low oestrogen OC used in the Spellacy experiments, will also cause a gentle suppression of the hypothalamic–pituitary axis.

Support for this concept comes from the experiments of Schneider *et al.*[24] who showed that serum LH levels remained the same as those found in the follicular phase under the influence of the triphasic preparation. That FSH was not suppressed is borne out by the levels of oestradiol-17β which also remained at the follicular level throughout the cycle, indicating that ovarian steroidogenesis was not completely arrested. However, it is obvious from the absence of the pre-ovulatory surge of oestrogen and LH that ovulation is blocked with the new triphasic.

With the triphasic, the presumed attenuated suppression, particularly in the first six days of treatment, is compensated for by a step-wise increase in the doses of EE and LNg in the next two phases where timing is important.

Figure 3.7 shows the relationship between normal ovarian and uterine changes and plasma oestrogen and progesterone levels throughout the ovulatory cycle of untreated women. The ovulatory cycle is divided into cycle days marked numerically from the onset of menses (day 1) onward in ascending order. At the bottom of Figure 3.7, the cycle is additionally divided into three phases: follicular, peri-ovulatory and luteal. In the normal ovulatory cycle, oestrogen levels gradually increase during the early follicular phase while progesterone levels remain extremely low. Drug administration is designed to coincide with these phases.

In Figure 3.8 the timing of the three-phase administration of the triphasic contraceptive is shown against the background of normal endocrine changes. The prescribed doses of EE and LNg and the time of administration during the cycle are superimposed over normal endogenous hormone levels.

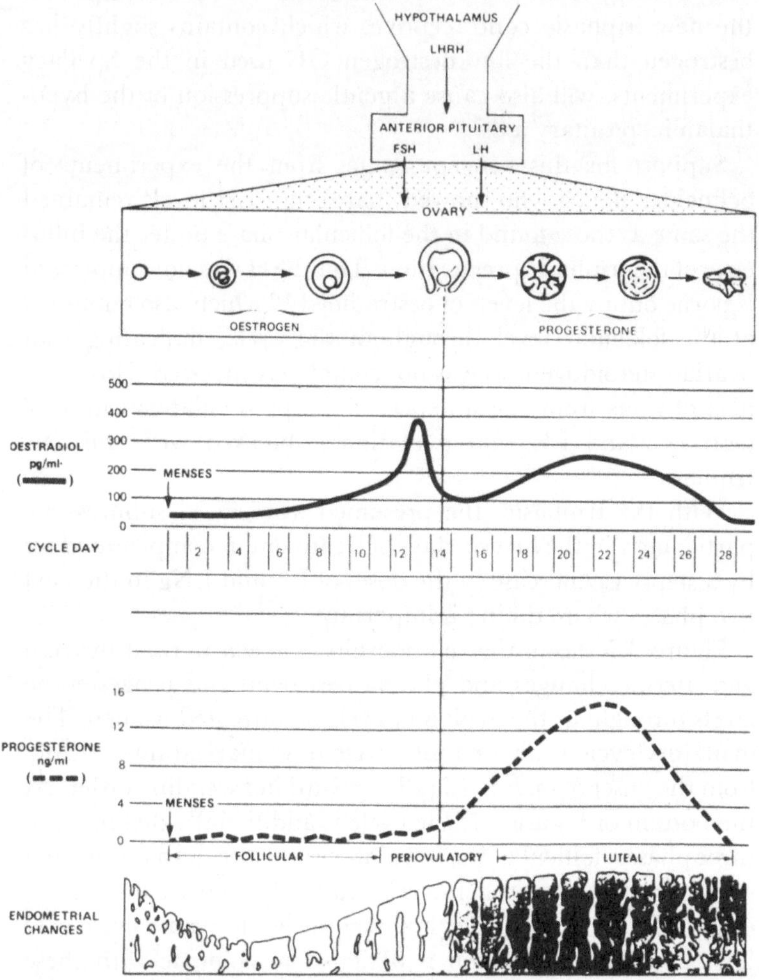

Figure 3.7 Diagram showing the hypothalamic–pituitary axis and the change induced by gonadotropin stimulation on the plasma levels of endogenous oestrogen and progesterone and the ovarian and endometrial changes during a normal menstrual cycle

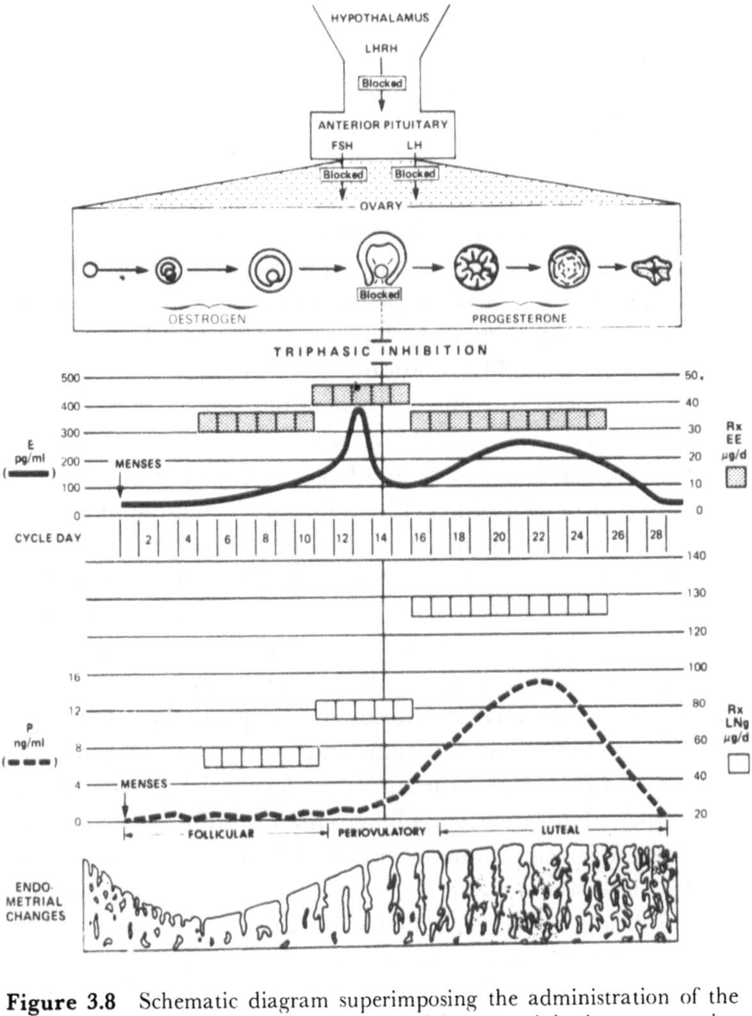

Figure 3.8 Schematic diagram superimposing the administration of the oestrogen and levonorgestrel components of the new triphasic contraceptive over a background of normal endogenous hormone levels. The three different steroid combinations are given in the follicular, peri-ovulatory and luteal phases at days in the cycle indicated in the figure, in dosages that mimic the rise and fall of normal hormonal changes

The first phase (early to mid-follicular) – 6 tablets of 30 μg EE plus 50 μg LNg – provides both low oestrogen and low progestagen. This dosage attempts to mimic follicular secretion necessary for promoting endometrial growth. Ovarian steroidogenesis is not completely arrested as shown by oestradiol levels similar to those found in the follicular phase[24].

In the second phase (peri-ovulatory) increased amounts of EE and LNg are provided in order to inhibit the LH surge and ovulation. Therefore, the next five tablets contain 40 μg EE plus 75 μg LNg. Both of these steroids in the quantities provided are known to inhibit ovulation when given alone. When given together, inhibition of ovulation is ensured. Thus a higher dose of LNg has been introduced earlier than the normal physiological time for progesterone increase.

The introduction of increased LNg levels just before the preovulatory surge of LH provides additional hypothalamic suppression. It may seem curious that exogenous oestrogen is being increased at this time since there is normally an endogenous preovulatory oestrogen surge. However, because this exogenous EE increase sufficiently precedes ovulation, this amount of EE will enhance the effect of LNg acting at the hypothalamic level to impede LHRH release, and on the pituitary, raising its threshold to hypothalamic stimulation and suppressing the LH surge. Most important, the increased levels of EE and LNg at this peri-ovulatory period will help maintain the endometrium and serve to lessen the chances of breakthrough bleeding and/or spotting that sometimes is observed with low dose formulations.

In addition, the increased levels of LNg increase the viscosity of the cervical mucus (cervical barrier), thereby increasing contraceptive protection by inhibiting the penetration of sperm.

The normal luteal phase is characterized by high progesterone levels. Oestrogen levels are lower than those found in the peri-ovulatory phase. The next 10 tablets administered in phase 3 are designed to mimic the luteal phase with 30 μg EE and 125 μg LNg in each tablet. These 10 tablets provide oestrogen and progestagen that would tend to mimic those being secreted by a functioning corpus luteum.

The seven-day tablet-free period that follows permits the exogenous steroid levels to decline and, consequently, withdrawal menstruation to occur. Again, this tablet-free interval mimics the physiological decline in steroid hormone that normally occurs.

A new, low-dose, effective three-phase preparation, providing a more physiological approach to contraception is now available.

CONCLUSION

The introduction of the triphasic approach represents an important contribution to contraceptive technology. The marked reduction in total steroid dose and maintenance of effective contraception is accomplished by taking advantage of the well-defined hormonal events during the normal cycle and superimposing upon this naturally fluctuating system the synergistic effects of levonorgestrel and ethinyloestradiol. The delivery of these steroids mimics the normal patterns of endogenous hormones during the menstrual cycle providing a more physiological approach to contraception.

A new, three-phase contraceptive preparation that maintains outstanding efficacy associated with a minimum of hormonal steroid is now available.

References

1. Beard, J., quoted by S. A. Asdell (1928). The growth and function of the corpus luteum. *Physiol. Rev.*, **8**, 313
2. Makepeace, A. W., Weinstein, G. L. and Friedman, M. H. (1937). The effect of progestin and progesterone on ovulation in the rabbit. *Am. J. Physiol.*, **119**, 512

3. Astwood, E. B. and Fevold, H. L. (1939). Action of progesterone on the gonadotropic activity of the pituitary. *Am. J. Physiol.*, **127**, 192
4. Rock, J., Pincus, G. and Garcia, C. R. (1956). Effects of certain 19-nor steroids on the human menstrual cycle. *Science*, **124**, 891
5. Rice-Wray, E. (1957). Field study with Enovid as a contraceptive agent. In *Proceedings of a Symposium on 19-Nor Progestational Steroids*, p. 78. (Chicago: Searle Research Laboratories)
6. Drill, V. A. (1966). *Oral Contraceptives.* (New York: McGraw-Hill)
7. Arnt, I. C., Ferrari, A., Sartoretto, J. N. and Woutersz, T. B. (1977). Low-dose combination oral contraceptives: A controlled clinical study of three different norgestrel–ethinyl estradiol ratios. *Fertil. Steril.*, **28**, 549
8. Goldzieher, J. W., De La Peña, A., Chenault, C. B. and Woutersz, T. B. (1975). Comparative studies of the ethynyl estrogens used in oral contraceptives. *Am. J. Obstet. Gynecol.*, **122**, 619
9. Spellacy, W. N., Kalra, P. S., Buhi, W. C. and Birk, S. A. (1980). Pituitary and ovarian responsiveness to a graded gonadotropin releasing factor stimulation test in women using a low-estrogen or a regular type of oral contraceptive. *Am. J. Obstet. Gynecol.*, **137**, 109
10. Kastin, A. J., Schally, A. V., Gual, C. and Arimura, A. (1972). Release of LH and FSH after administration of synthetic LH-releasing hormone. *J. Clin. Endocrinol. Metab.*, **34**, 753
11. Kastin, A. J., Gual, C. and Schally, A. V. (1972). Clinical experience with hypothalamic releasing hormones. Part 2. Luteinizing hormone-releasing hormone and other hypophysiotropic releasing hormones. *Recent Prog. Horm. Res.*, **28**, 201
12. Vandenberg, G., DeVane, G. and Yen, S. S. C. (1974). Effects of exogenous estrogen and progestin on pituitary responsiveness to synthetic luteinizing hormone-releasing factor. *J. Clin. Invest.*, **53**, 1750
13. Schally, A. V., Locke, W., Kastin, A. J. and Bowers, C. Y. (1967–68). *Yearbook of Endocrinology*, **5**
14. Mishell, Jr., D. R., Kletzky, O. A., Brenner, P. F., Roy, S. and Nicoloff, J. (1977). The effect of contraceptive steroids on hypothalamic-pituitary function. *Am. J. Obstet. Gynecol.*, **128**, 60
15. Scott, J. Z., Kletzky, O. A., Brenner, P. F. and Mishell, D. R. (1978). Comparison of the effects of contraceptive steroid formulations containing two doses of estrogen on pituitary function. *Fertil. Steril.*, **30**, 141
16. Robyn, C., Schöndorf, H., Jürgenson, O., Dericks-Tan, J. S. E. and Taubert, H.-D. (1974). Oral contraception can decrease the pituitary capacity to release gonadotropins in response to synthetic LH-releasing hormone. *Arch. Gynaekol.*, **216**, 73
17. Perez-Lopez, F. R., L'Hermite, M. and Robyn, C. (1975). Gonadotropin hormone releasing tests in women receiving hormonal contraception. *Clin. Endocrinol.*, **4**, 477
18. Krög, W., Aktories, K., Dericks-Tan, J. S. E. and Taubert, H.-D. (1976). Dose dependent inhibition by oral contraceptives of the pituitary to

release LH and FSH in response to stimulation with LH-RH. *Contraception*, **15**, 171

19. Beattie, C. W. and Corbin, A. (1975). The differential effects of diestrous progestogen administration on proestrous gonadotrophin levels. *Endocrinology*, **97**, 885
20. Moghissi, K. S. and Marks, C. (1971). Effects of microdose norgestrel on endogenous gonadotropic and steroid hormones, cervical mucus properties, vaginal cytology, and endometrium. *Fertil. Steril.*, **22**, 424
21. Johansson, E. D. B. (1973). Studies of compounds that interfere with the normal function of the corpus luteum in women. *Excerpta Med. Int. Congr. Ser.*, **278**, 276
22. Roland, M., Leisten, D. and Caruso, L. J. (1973). A cyclic progestagen regimen for fertility control. *Excerpta Med. Int. Congr. Ser.*, **278**, 265
23. Moghissi, K. S. (1973). Effects of microdose progestogens on endogenous gonadotrophic and steroid hormones, cervical mucus properties, vaginal cytology and endometrium. *Excerpta Med. Int. Congr. Ser.*, **278**, 260
24. Schneider, W. H. F., Spona, J., Schmid, R. and Lachnit-Fixson, U. (1977). Efficacy of three-phase oral contraceptives. *Excerpta Med. Int. Congr. Ser.*, **441**, 126
25. Corbin, A. (1979). Contraceptive technology in the future. In Briggs, M. H. and Corbin, A. (eds.) *Advances in Steroid Biochemistry and Pharmacology*, Vol. 7, pp. 1–8. (London: Academic Press)

4
Mode of action of triphasic oral contraception

J. SPONA, W. H. F. SCHNEIDER and
U. LACHNIT-FIXSON

ABSTRACT

The present experiments were carried out to investigate the borderline dose for inhibition of ovulation by levonorgestrel and to study the mode of action of triphasic oral contraception. The borderline dose for inhibition of ovulation was found to be 50 μg levonorgestrel per day. In addition, bioavailability of levonorgestrel after daily oral administration of 50 μg and 100 μg, respectively, was recorded between 400 and 600 pg/ml serum. Daily ingestion of 150 μg levonorgestrel resulted in serum levels of 1 ng/ml. Two different preparations of a triphasic oral contraceptive were studied. The test preparations of a triphasic oral composition: SH B 264 AB: six coated tablets containing 30 μg of ethinyloestradiol and 50 μg of levonorgestrel; five coated tablets containing 40 μg of ethinyloestradiol and 75 μg of levonorgestrel; and ten coated tablets containing 30 μg of ethinyloestradiol and 125 μg of levonorgestrel. SH B 261 AB: six coated tablets containing 30 μg of ethinyloestradiol and 50 μg of levonorgestrel; five coated tablets containing 50 μg of ethinyloestradiol and 50 μg of levonorgestrel; and ten coated tablets containing 40 μg ethinyloestradiol and 125 μg of levonorgestrel.

Serum levels of LH, 17β-oestradiol and progesterone were estimated by radioimmunoassay in five women receiving either SH B 264 AB or SH B 261 AB. In addition, the cervical score and the karyopyknotic index of vaginal smear samples were recorded. The data of the present investigation combine to suggest that triphasic oral contraception by SH B 264 AB acts by inhibiting ovulation and by providing a back-up mechanism by reducing the cervical score. The reduction of levonorgestrel dose in SH B 264 AB does not interfere with cycle control, since the triphasic oral contraceptive very precisely mimics endogenous sex hormone serum levels of the normal cycle. Thus, patterns of endometrial hormone-receptor levels similar to those found in normal cycles are to be expected. The present preparation of this new generation of oral contraceptives is a well-balanced formulation providing greatest contraceptive safety and the least side-effects possible.

INTRODUCTION

Recent retrospective[1–6] and prospective[7] studies have shown that oral contraceptives may cause unwanted side-effects. Attention has been focused on possible risks of oestrogen-dependent metabolic complications such as thromboembolic diseases, neurovascular accidents, myocardial infarctions, abnormal carbohydrate metabolism, lipid metabolism and biliary cholestasis. A positive correlation between oestrogen dose of ovulation inhibitors and the frequency of thromboembolic diseases was registered upon statistical analysis of data[1–7]. On the other hand, oestrogens were noted to favourably influence high density lipoprotein (HDL) serum levels, whereas progestagens derived from 19-nortestosterone type derivatives were reported to reduce HDL concentrations in blood[8].

Previous experience had shown that oral contraceptives with an oestrogen content of 50 μg of ethinyloestradiol per day and a progestagen content varying in accordance with the two-phase principle afforded as much contraceptive security as classical single-phase oral contraceptives of the combined type[9,10]. Such sequential-type oral contraceptives allowed reduction of the progestagen dose. In addition, adaption of the progestin dose to the phases of the normal cycle rendered it possible to bring about cyclic alterations of the endometrium (11) and vaginal epithelium (10), such as those noted in normal menstrual cycles.

The aim of the present investigation was to study the borderline dose of ovulation inhibition by levonorgestrel*.

In addition, it was the purpose of the present study to investigate the mode of action of the first three-phase type of oral contraceptives, which allows the administration of the oestrogen and progestagen according to the patterns of serum levels noted in normal cycles. The results of clinical trials using this new generation of oral contraceptives were reported recently[12,13].

MATERIAL AND METHODS

The ovulation-inhibiting dose of levonorgestrel was determined in a total of 12 women between 20 and 28 years of age with normal cycles. Following a control cycle, they were treated from the fifth to the 25th day of the cycle with daily oral doses of 30, 50, 100 or 150 μg of levonorgestrel. Starting on the eighth day of the cycle, they were subjected to daily examinations of the karyopyknotic index and cervical score[14] as well as to radioimmunological estimation of the serum levels of luteinizing hormone (LH), follicle-stimulating hormone (FSH), progesterone (P) and oestradiol (E_2)[15]. In addition, 12 hours after ingestion of levonorgestrel, its serum level was determined by the radioimmunological technique described by Spona *et al.* [16]. Results of radioimmunoassays were evaluated by a computer program[17] on a PDP-8/e computer.

* Levonorgestrel and D-norgestrel are used synonymously throughout this paper.

On the basis of radioimmunoassay data, the cycles could be classified as follows: normal cycle, luteal insufficiency, follicular maturation and inhibition of ovulation. Luteal insufficiency was defined by progesterone serum levels below 3.0 ng/ml.

The test preparations had the following compositions: SH B 264 AB: six coated tablets containing 30 μg of ethinyloestradiol and 50 μg of levonorgestrel; five coated tablets containing 40 μg of ethinyloestradiol and 75 μg of levonorgestrel; and ten coated tablets containing 30 μg of ethinyloestradiol and 125 μg of levonorgestrel. SH B 261 AB: six coated tablets containing 30 μg of ethinyloestradiol and 50 μg of levonorgestrel; five coated tablets containing 50 μg of ethinyloestradiol and 50 μg of levonorgestrel; and ten coated tablets containing 40 μg of ethinyloestradiol and 125 μg of levonorgestrel. This implies that the ten-day imitation of a 'luteal phase', which has proved so successful in the two-phase preparation SH 71172, is maintained, while the 'follicular phase' (just as in the normal cycle) is subdivided into a post-menstrual and a peri-ovulatory phase. The investigation was carried out in ten female volunteers, aged between 22 and 26 years, who were subdivided at random into two test groups of five women, receiving either SH B 264 AB or SH B 261 AB. During the first test cycle the test preparations were administered from the first day of the cycle, and the usual seven-day tablet-free intervals were allowed between subsequent administrations. All parameters of cyclic function were determined continuously during a control cycle prior to the investi-

Table 4.1 Set-up of experiments on mode of action of SH B 261 AB and SH B 264 AB. × indicates the cycles investigated

Preparation	*Number of subjects*	*Control cycle*	*First treatment cycle*	*Second treatment cycle*	*Third treatment cycle*	*Control cycle*
SH B 264 AB	5	×	×	—	×	×
SH B 261 AB	5	×	×	—	×	×

gation to make sure ovulation occurred, again during the first and third cycles during administration of the test preparations and, finally, during one cycle without treatment. A survey of the cycles studied is given in Table 4.1.

The levels of LH refer to the LER 907 standard and were recorded in mIU/ml serum; the levels of oestradiol were recorded in pg/ml serum and those of progesterone in ng/ml serum. Blood samples were always drawn at the same time of the day, approximately 12 hours after administration. Dr Hartmann (Schering AG, Berlin, GFR) was kind enough to carry out the statistical calculations for the mean value curves.

RESULTS

Administrations of different doses of levonorgestrel only suggest that the borderline dose for inhibition of ovulation is 50 μg per day (Table 4.2). The daily administration of 30 μg of levonorgestrel was found to cause luteal insufficiency (Figure 4.1) in one subject and follicular maturation (Figure 4.2) in two females out of four subjects. In one test subject a completely normal cycle occurred. Doses greater than 50 μg of levonorgestrel were noted to inhibit ovulation (Table 4.2).

The bioavailability of levonorgestrel after daily oral administrations of doses between 30 and 150 μg is depicted in Figure

Table 4.2 Ovulation inhibition by levonorgestrel. The evaluation of cycles and of borderline dose was carried out as described under Materials and Methods

Dose (μg)	*Number of subjects*	*Inhibition of ovulation*	*Follicular maturation*	*Luteal insufficiency*	*Normal cycle*
30	4	—	2	1	1
50	3	2	1	—	—
100	3	3	—	—	—
150	2	2	—	—	—

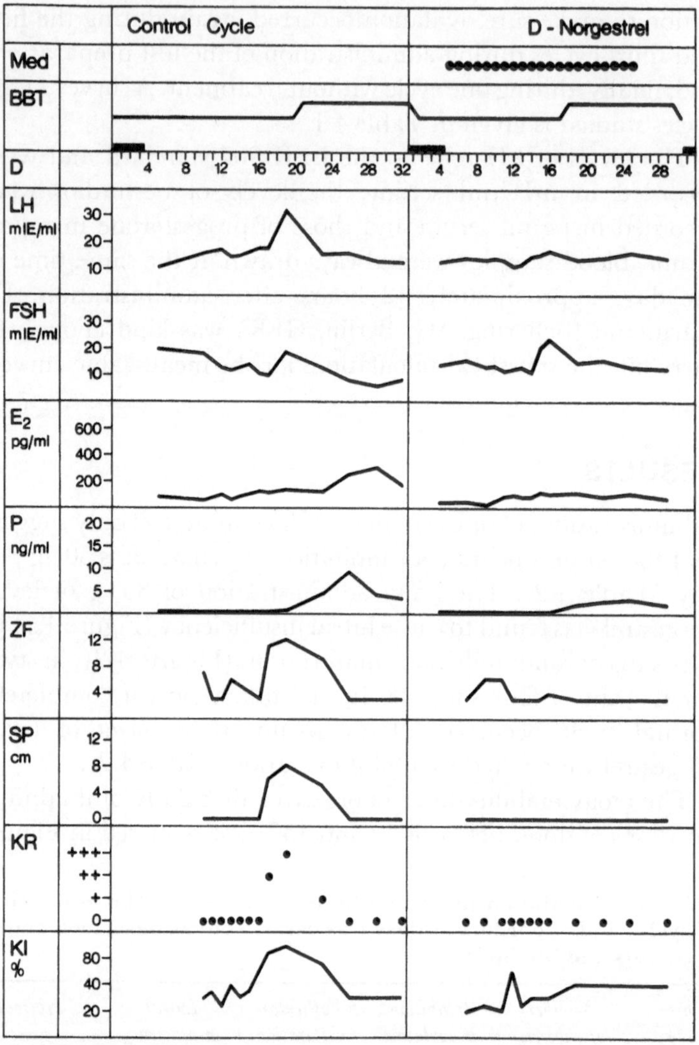

Figure 4.1 Hormone serum levels, cervical score and karyopyknotic index before and during the daily treatment of the subject with 30 μg of levonorgestrel. The treatment was found to cause luteal insufficiency in this particular female. Luteal insufficiency was judged by serum levels below 3.0 ng/ml

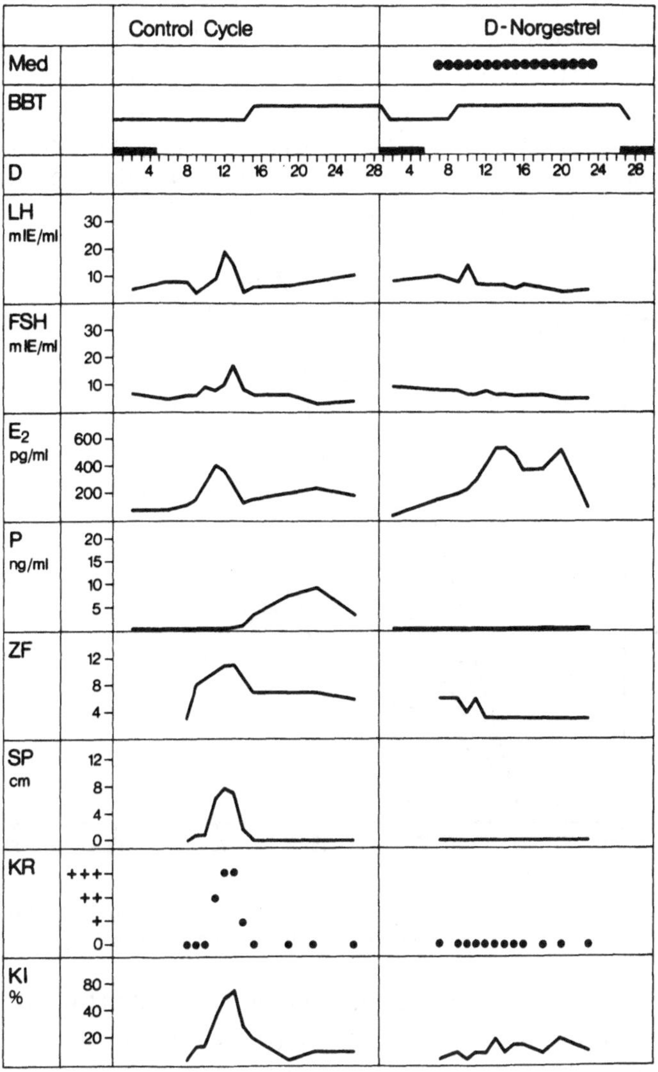

Figure 4.2 Serum levels of hormones, cervical score and karyopyknotic index in one subject before and during daily treatment with 30 μg of levonorgestrel

4.3. The serum levels of levonorgestrel were recorded to be quite similar after the ingestion of 50 and 100 μg, respectively. Levonorgestrel serum levels varied between 400 and 600 pg/ml after either dose. The administration of 30 μg of levonorgestrel resulted in serum levels of some 200 pg/ml. A pronounced rise in the bioavailability was registered when the dose of levonorgestrel was increased to 150 μg (Figure 4.3).

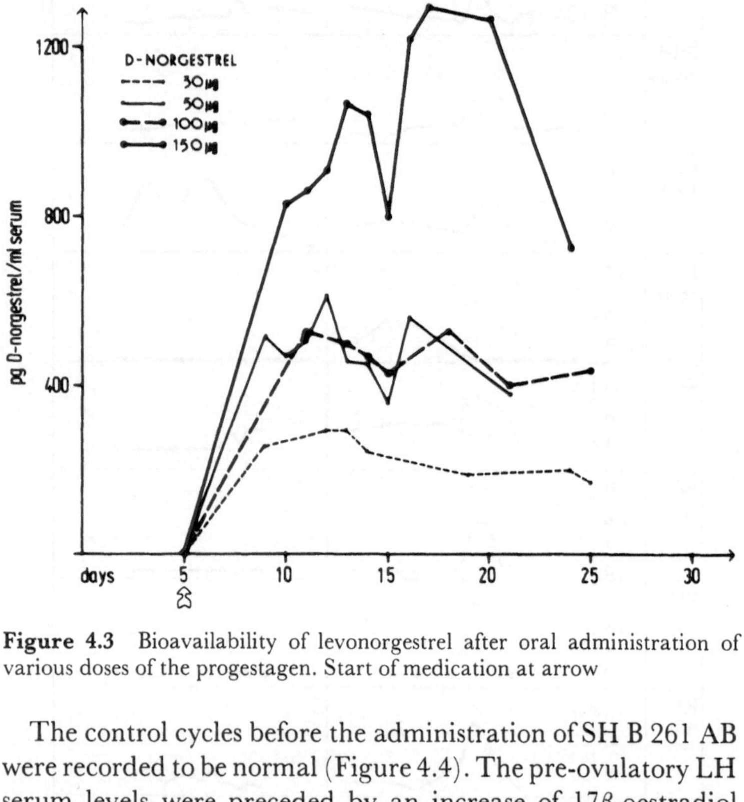

Figure 4.3 Bioavailability of levonorgestrel after oral administration of various doses of the progestagen. Start of medication at arrow

The control cycles before the administration of SH B 261 AB were recorded to be normal (Figure 4.4). The pre-ovulatory LH serum levels were preceded by an increase of 17β-oestradiol levels, which indicated follicular activity. A concomitant rise in oestrogenic activity was noted as reflected by the cervical and karyopyknotic index. All peripheral parameters decreased upon

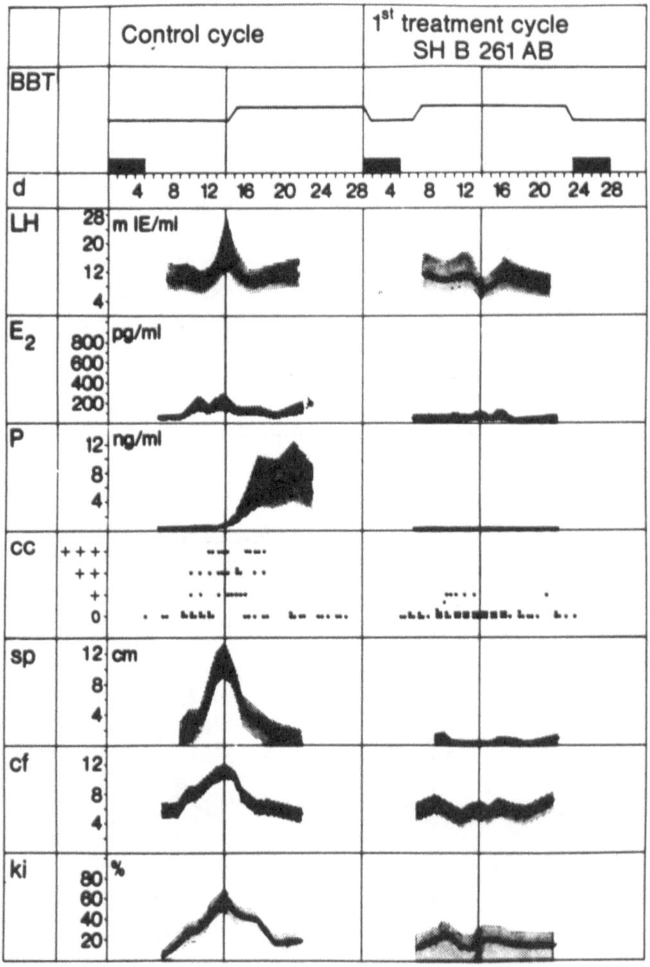

Figure 4.4 Serum levels of hormones, cervical score and karyopyknotic index, before and during the first treatment cycle in five subjects with SH B 261 AB. Results are given as means ± SD. BBT = basal body temperature; E2 = 17β-oestradiol; P = progesterone; cc = crystallization capacity; sp = spinnbarkeit; cf = cervical score; ki = karyopyknotic index

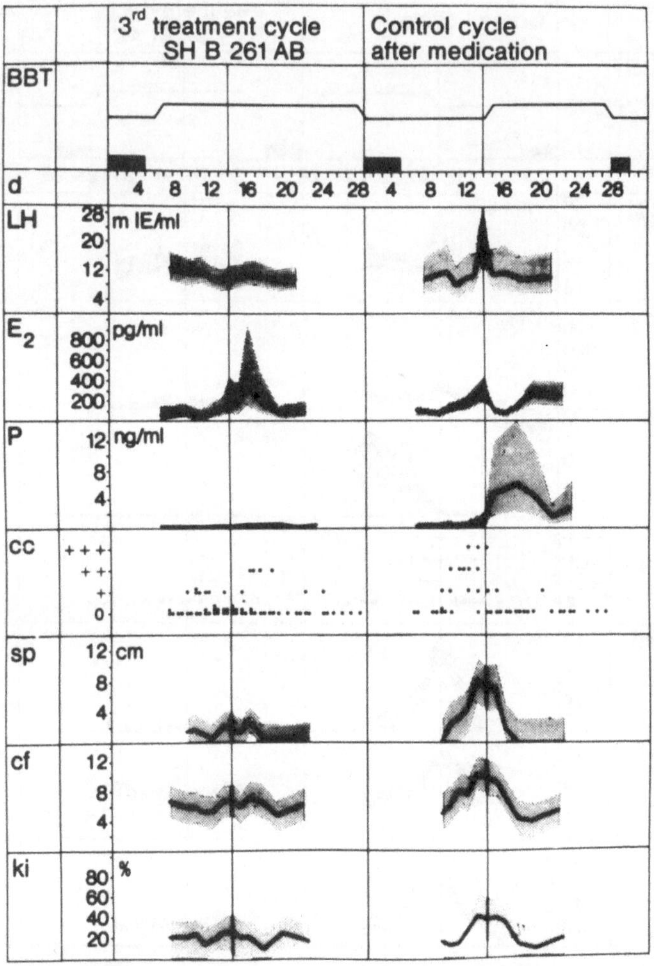

Figure 4.5 Serum levels of LH, 17β-oestradiol and progesterone, cervical score and karyopyknotic index in five females during the third treatment cycle and after discontinuation of treatment with SH B 261 AB. Abbreviations as Figure 4.4

the increase of progesterone serum levels, and a normal luteal phase was observed in all subjects. During the first cycle of treatment with SH B 261 AB anovulatory cycles were registered in all females (Figure 4.4). Additionally, suppression of cervical score and karyopyknotic index was recorded. During the third SH B 261 AB treatment cycle LH serum levels remained low and no peak values were noted (Figure 4.5). But, 17β-oestradiol serum levels rose to pre-ovulatory values in three out of five females at midcycle and remained elevated until day 20 of the cycle (Figure 4.4). Concomitantly, an increase of cervical scores was found. The karyopyknotic index, on the other hand, did not show such a pronounced increase. In one of the test subjects, together with the increase in oestradiol levels, the serum progesterone levels also rose but stayed far below the lowest limits indicative of an ovulatory cycle. During all treatment cycles of all subjects very good cycle control and tolerance was noted. All subjects exhibited normal ovulatory cycles during the subsequent control cycles.

Cycles were found to be ovulatory in all subjects prior to treatment with SH B 264 AB. Inhibition of ovulation was observed in all five females during the treatment with SH B 264 AB (Figure 4.6). Serum LH concentrations remained at low levels of the early follicular phase indicating that central inhibition was operative. In addition, a uniform pattern of 17β-oestradiol serum levels was recorded, and no midcycle rise was observed. A concomitant reduction of the cervical score was found. Spinnbarkeit and crystallization capacity of the cervical secretion was markedly reduced. The karyopyknotic index fluctuated and reached a maximum of about 25% as compared to some 65% in ovulatory cycles at midcycle (Figure 4.6). Similarly, inhibition of all parameters of cyclic function was noted in all five subjects during the third cycle of treatment with SH B 264 AB (Figure 4.7). Withdrawal bleeding was on average on the third day after discontinuation of treatment in this group of patients. No spotting or breakthrough bleeding was observed.

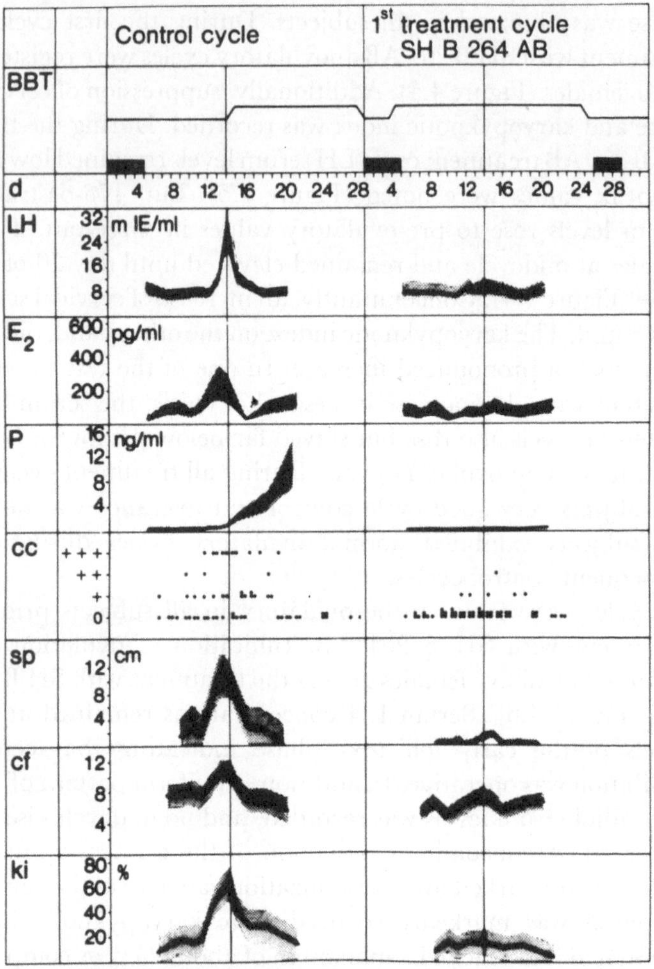

Figure 4.6 Monitoring of hormone serum levels, cervical score and karyopyknotic index in five females prior to and during treatment with SH B 264 AB. Abbreviations as Figure 4.4

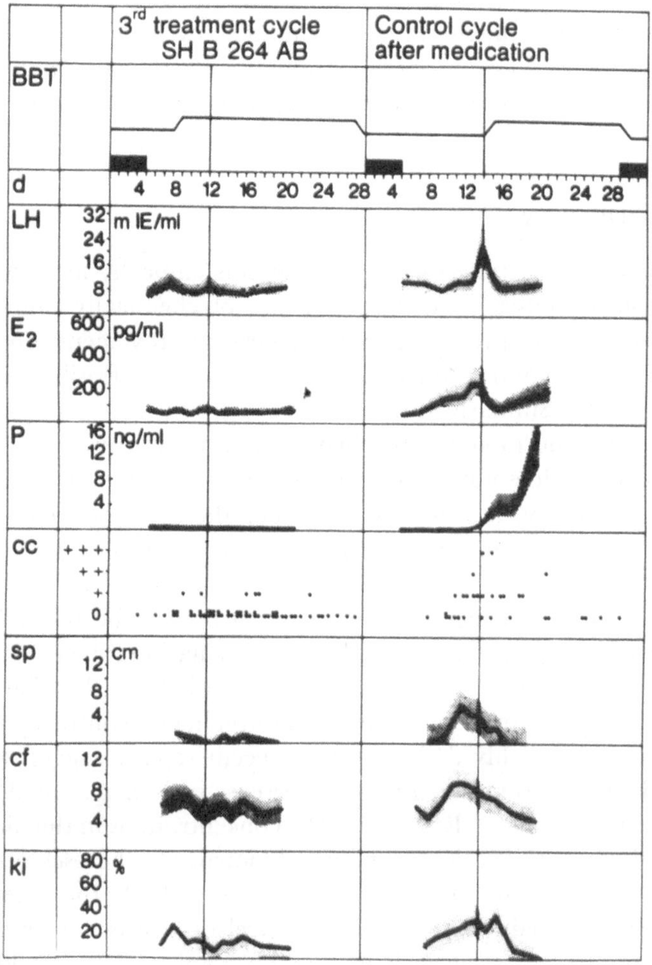

Figure 4.7 Parameters of cyclic function during the third cycle of administration and the control cycle after discontinuation of SH B 264 AB. Abbreviations as Figure 4.4

Monitoring of hormone serum levels after discontinuation of SH B 264 AB treatment revealed ovulatory cycles in all subjects (Figure 4.7). The peripheral parameters, on the other hand, as yet did not reflect the return of complete functional activity.

DISCUSSION

It takes a long time to test new steroids clinically for contraceptive purposes. Therefore, the use of chemically different oestrogens and progestagens to achieve improvements on the present oral contraceptives does not appear to be feasible in the near future. Similarly, introduction of contraceptive procedures other than hormonal or biochemical methods as discussed previously[18–20] does not seem to be possible at present. An alternative possibility, therefore, is to reduce the doses of oestrogens and/or progestagens which are currently used in oral contraceptives.

The present experiments clearly show that the borderline dose of levonorgestrel for inhibition of ovulation is below 50 μg when administered daily over 21 days (Table 4.2). The reduction of the total dose of levonorgestrel in oral contraceptives seems to be highly desirable since recent reports suggest that HDL cholesterol concentrations decrease with increasing doses of progestagen[21–23]. Reduced HDL concentrations in the blood are thought to accelerate the development of atherosclerosis[24] by impairing the clearance of cholesterol from the arterial wall[25,26]. A reduction of levonorgestrel dosage is not feasible beyond the 150 μg level when using it in combination with 30 μg ethinyloestradiol in a conventional fixed-dose schedule throughout the cycle due to an expected poor cycle control. An improvement on previous oral contraceptives was achieved by mimicking the endogenous levels of oestrogen and progestagen during a normal menstrual cycle. This sequential type of oral contraceptives (biphasic)[9] allowed reduction of the prostagen dose by

43%, but contained 60% more oestrogen than the combined type of oral contraceptive with lowest oestrogen content (150/30). Oestrogens, on the other hand, were reported to cause a great many undesirable side-effects[1–7].

Previous experience with a 30 μg ethinyloestradiol formulation of oral contraceptive[27] and the knowledge of the borderline dose of levonorgestrel for inhibition of ovulation being below 50 μg (Table 4.2) prompted the development of a triphasic type of sequential oral contraceptive[12]. This three-phase

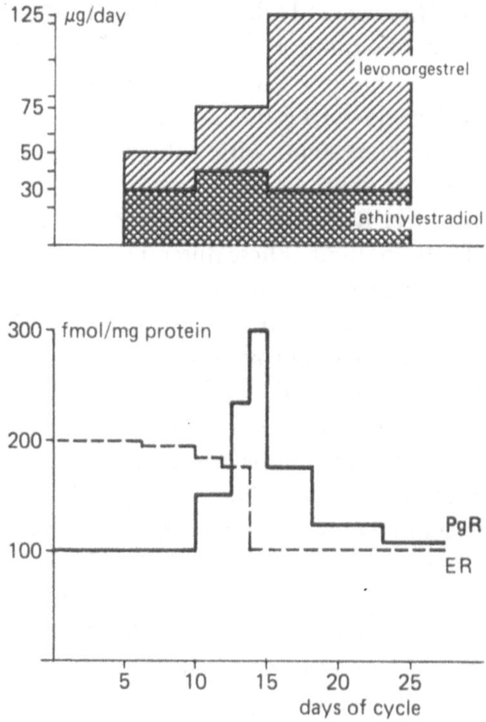

Figure 4.8 Schematic presentation of staggered dosage of oestrogen and progestagen during treatment with SH B 264 AB and oestrogen-receptor (ER) as well as progesterone-receptor (PgR) levels in the endometrium during a normal cycle[28]

sequential type allows us to mimic more precisely the endogenous levels of 17β-oestradiol and progesterone in normal menstrual cycles. This first type of the new generation of oral contraceptives combines the advantage of providing an improved cycle control with reduction of undesirable side-effects[12,13].

Data regarding the serum levels of levonorgestrel suggest no great differences in bioavailability when administered in 50 and 100 μg doses (Figure 4.3). These results are in agreement with experiments on the ovulation inhibition dose (Table 4.2).

It was interesting to note that some differences emerged from the comparison between SH B 264 AB with SH B 261 AB. Perfect inhibition of ovulation was noted during the treatment with SH B 264 AB (Figures 4.6 and 4.7). However, patterns of hormone serum levels during the treatment with SH B 261 AB (Figure 4.5) are consistent with follicular maturation. In addition, a small rise of progesterone serum levels in one subject during the third SH B 261 AB treatment cycle suggests luteal insufficiency in this patient. These differences may be caused by the slightly smaller progestagen dosage of SH B 261 AB.

The present data combine to suggest that SH B 264 AB acts by inhibiting ovulation and providing a back-up mechanism by reducing the cervical score. The reduction of the levonorgestrel dose in SH B 264 AB does not interfere with cycle control. This is the result of very precisely mimicking sex steroid serum levels of the normal menstrual cycle. Thus, presumably similar endometrial oestrogen-receptor (ER) and progesterone-receptor (PgR) levels are obtained in SH B 264 AB treated subjects compared to subjects with normal menstrual cycles (Figure 4.8). Such fluctuating patterns of ER and PgR levels (Figure 4.8) are of importance for a good cycle control and for prevention of possible nidation of fertilized eggs.

The present preparation of this new generation of oral contraceptives is a well-balanced formulation providing the greatest contraceptive safety and the least side-effects possible.

Acknowledgements

We greatly appreciate a gift of LER 907 from the National Institute of Arthritis, Metabolism and Digestive Diseases which was used as LH standard in our radioimmunoassay work. We are grateful to Dr A. S. Hartree for providing us with highly purified LH, which was used to prepare the tracer for the LH assay. We thank Mrs J. Adolph for help during the preparation of the manuscript.

References

1. Collaborative Group for the Study of Stroke in Young Women (1975). Oral contraceptives and stroke in young women. *J. Am. Med. Assoc.*, **231**, 718
2. Collaborative Group for the Study of Stroke in Young Women (1973). Oral contraception and increased risk of cerebral ischemia or thrombosis. *N. Engl. J. Med.*, **288**, 871
3. Mann, J. I., Vessey, M. P., Thorogood, M. and Doll, R.(1975). Myocardial infarction in young women with special reference to oral contraceptive practice. *Br. Med. J.*, **2**, 241
4. Mann, J. I. and Inman, W. H. W. (1975). Oral contraceptives and death from myocardial infarction. *Br. Med. J.*, **2**, 245
5. Vessey, M. P., Doll, R., Fairnbairn, A. S. and Glober, E. (1970). Postoperative thromboembolism and the use of oral contraceptives. *Br. Med. J.*, **2**, 123
6. Boston Collaborative Drug Surveillance Program (1973). Oral contraceptives and venous thromboembolic disease, surgically confirmed gallbladder disease and breast tumors. *Lancet*, **1**, 1399
7. Royal College of General Practitioners (1974). *Oral Contraceptives and Health.* (New York: Pitman Publishing Comp.)
8. Briggs, M. and Briggs, M. (1978). *Oral Contraceptives*, **2**, p. 87 (Edinburgh: Churchill Livingstone)
9. Lachnit-Fixson, U. (1975). Einführung und weitere Ergebnisse zur klinischen Prüfung von Sequilar®. *Med. Mitt. (Schering)*, **5**
10. Schneider, W. H. F., Schmid, R. and Spona, J. (1975). Über das Wirkungsspektrum von Sequilar®. *Med. Mitt. (Schering)*, **5**, 5
11. Brosens, I., Robertson, W. B. and van Assche, A. (1975). Endometrium-Befunde unter Anwendung eines neuen D-norgestrelhaltigen Zweistufenpräparates. *Med. Mitt. (Schering)*, **5**, 9
12. Lachnit-Fixson, U. (1979). Erstes Dreistufenpräparat zur hormonalen Konzeptionsverhütung. *Münch. Med. Wochenschr.*, **121**, 1419

13. Zador, G. (1979). Fertility regulation using triphasic administration of ethinyl estradiol and laevenorgestrel in comparison with the 30 plus 150 μg fixed dose regime. *Acta Obstet. Gynecol. Scand. Suppl.* **88**, 43
14. Spona, J. and Schneider, W. H. F. (1976). Central and peripheral parameters of the menstrual cycle under the influence of a new combined oral contraceptive. *Acta Obstet. Gynecol. Scand. Suppl.*, **54**, 45
15. Gitsch, E., Schneider, W. H. F. and Spona, J. (1977). Radioimmunoassay. In E. Gitsch (ed.). *Radioisotope in Geburtshilfe und Gynäkologie*, p. 373. (Berlin: Walter de Gryuter)
16. Spona, J., Weiner, E., Nieuweboer, B., Hümpel, M., Schneider, W. H. F. and Johansson, E. D. B. (1977). Injectable depot contraceptives on D-Norgestrel basis II. Clinical pharmacokinetic studies with D-Norgestrel undecylate in women. *Contraception*, **15**, 413
17. Spona, J. (1974). Rapid assay of LH and evaluation of data by new computer program. In *RIA and Related Procedures in Medicine*. (Vienna: International Atomic Energy Agency)
18. Hawkins, D. F. and Elder, M. G. (1979). *Human Fertility Control*. (London, Boston: Butterworths)
19. Diamond, M. C. and Korenbrot, C. C. (1978). *Hormonal Contraceptives, Estrogens and Human Welfare*. (New York, London: Academic Press)
20. Briggs, M. H. and Briggs, M. (1976). *Biochemical Contraception*. (New York, London: Academic Press)
21. Bradley, D. D., Wingerd, J., Petitti, D. B., Kraus, R. M. and Ramcharan, S. (1978). Serum HDL-cholesterol in women using oral contraceptives estrogens and progestins. *N. Engl. J. Med.*, **299**, 17
22. Larsson-Cohn, U., Wallentin, L. and Zador, G. (1979). Plasma lipids and HDL during oral contraception with different combinations of ethinylestradiol and levonorgestrel. *Horm. Metab. Res.*, **11**, 437
23. Rössner, S. (1978). Lowering of HDL cholesterol by oral contraceptives. *Lancet*, **2**, 269
24. Jenkins, P. J., Harper, R. W. and Nestel, P. J. (1978). Severity of coronary atherosclerosis related to lipoprotein concentration. *Br. Med. J.*, **2**, 388
25. Miller, G. I. and Miller, N. E. (1975). HDL concentration and development of ischemic heart disease. *Lancet*, **1**, 16
26. Miller, N. E., Porde, O. H. and Thelle, D. S. (1977). The Thromso heart study: HDL and coronary heart disease: A prospective case control study. *Lancet*, **1**, 965
27. Zador, G. and Nilsson, B. (1977). Clinical experience with a low-estrogen, low-progestagen combined oral contraceptive. Evaluation of a Swedish multicentre study. *Pharmatherapeutica*, **1**, 453
28. Spona, J., Ulm, R., Bieglmayer, C. and Husslein, P. (1979). Hormone serum levels and hormone receptor contents of endometria in women with normal menstrual cycles and patients bearing endometrial carcinoma. *Gynecol. Obstet. Invest.*, **10**, 71

5
Effects of some ethinyloestradiol/levonorgestrel combinations on SHBG and on lipid metabolism

U. LARSSON-COHN, L. FÅHREUS, L. WALLENTIN and G. ZADOR

In Western societies the mortality from cardiovascular disease is some 6–7 times higher in males than in females in the age group between 40 and 50 years. It can thus be suspected that besides well established risk factors such as plasma lipid levels, age, overweight, diabetes, hypertension, smoking etc., the gender may also be of importance for the development of atherosclerosis. This is why our group has for some years been interested in the influence of sexual hormones on the lipid status.

Although the plasma concentrations of cholesterol and triglycerides are well established as being positively correlated to the risk for cardiovascular disease, it has in later years become evident that the pattern of the lipoproteins is of much greater significance in this context. In recent years both experimental and epidemiological studies have shown that a low HDL level probably is one of the most potent risk factors for atherosclerotic cardiovascular disease[1,2]. In order to obtain a meaningful picture of the lipid effects of a therapeutic agent it is therefore not sufficient to measure only the plasma concentrations of cholesterol and triglycerides. In some situations the total plasma cholesterol may remain unchanged while the cholesterol within the HDL, the 'good cholesterol', may change significantly. The ratio between HDL-cholesterol and total plasma cholesterol seems to be the lipoprotein parameter that is considered the best risk indicator for ischaemic cardiovascular disease.

MATERIAL AND METHODS

Ninety-eight women seeking contraceptive advice were randomly allocated into 4 treatment groups, each group receiving one of four different combined oral contraceptive drugs. The drugs are specified in Table 5.1.

Fasting blood samples were collected twice before treatment and on one of the last treatment days of cycles 1, 3 and 6. The lipids were measured using standard methods including the precipitation technique for assay of HDL. SHBG was measured by Dr E. O. B. Johansson, Uppsala, Sweden. All statistical differences were calculated on values obtained by each treatment value being expressed as a percentage of the mean of the corresponding pretreatment values.

Table 5.1 Composition of the four drugs that were used

Drug	*Ethinyloestradiol (EE) (μg)*	*Levonorgestrel (LNg) (μg)*	*EE : LNg ratio*
20/250	30	250	0.08
30/250	30	250	0.12
30/150	30	150	0.2
Triphasic 6 × 30/50 + 5 × 40/75 + 10 × 30/125			0.35

RESULTS

The detailed results of this study will be published elsewhere. Figures 5.1–5.4 show the results from the determinations of SHBG, triglycerides, cholesterol and HDL-cholesterol.

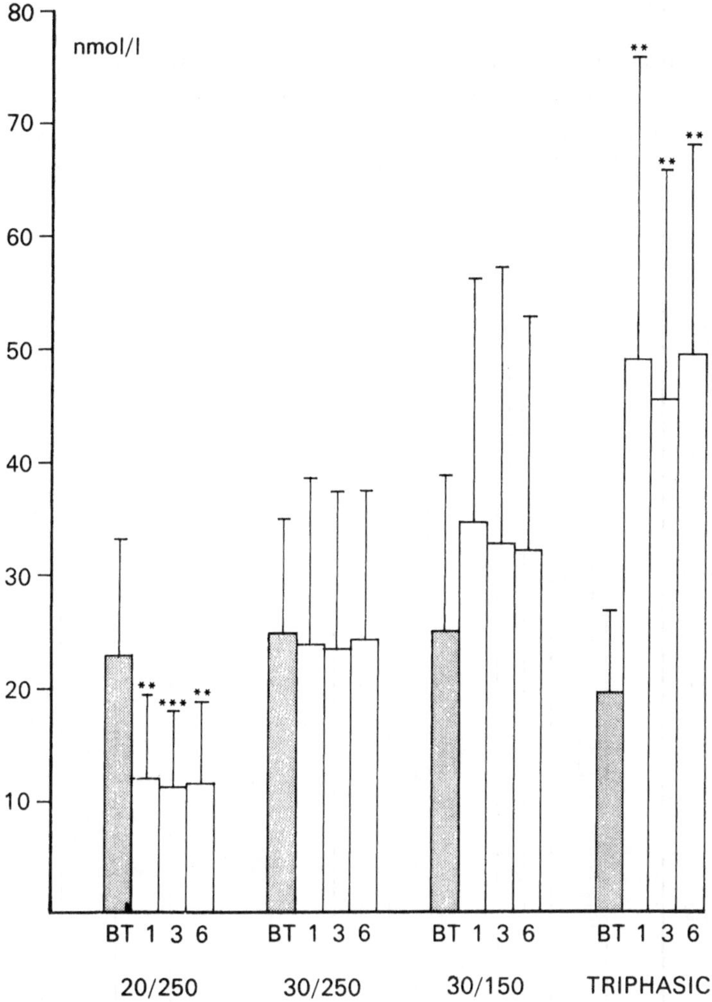

Figure 5.1 The influence of four different combined oral contraceptives on SHBG concentrations in plasma (mean ± SD). BT = before treatment; 1 = after one month of treatment; 3 = after three months of treatment; 6 = after six months of treatment.
* = $p < 0.05$; ** = $p < 0.01$; *** = $p < 0.001$

SHBG

In all treatment groups SHBG reached a stable level already during the first month of treatment. After six months the mean concentration was reduced 41% by 20/250 and unchanged by 30/250 while there was a moderate and statistically insignificant

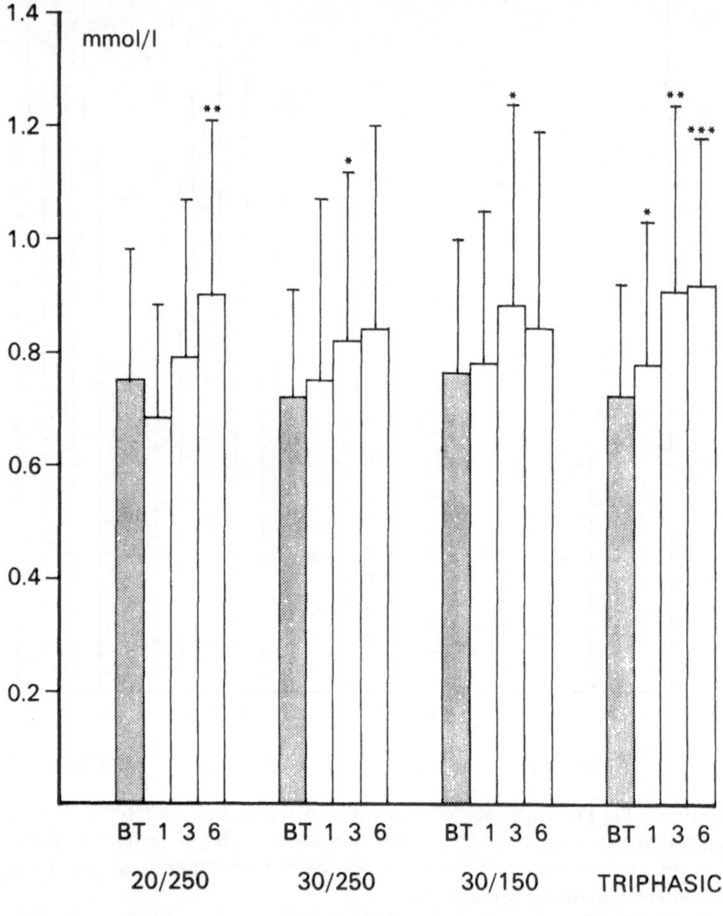

Figure 5.2 The influence of four different combined oral contraceptives on triglyceride concentrations in plasma (mean ± SD). Key as in Figure 5.1

increase by 30/150 and a marked increase (202%) by the triphasic drug. After six months the coefficient of correlation between the mean changes of SHBG and the EE/LNg ratios was 0.997.

Cholesterol

The concentration of total cholesterol was lowered in the subjects taking 20/250, 30/250 or 30/150 after one month but not after three or six months. No other changes appeared.

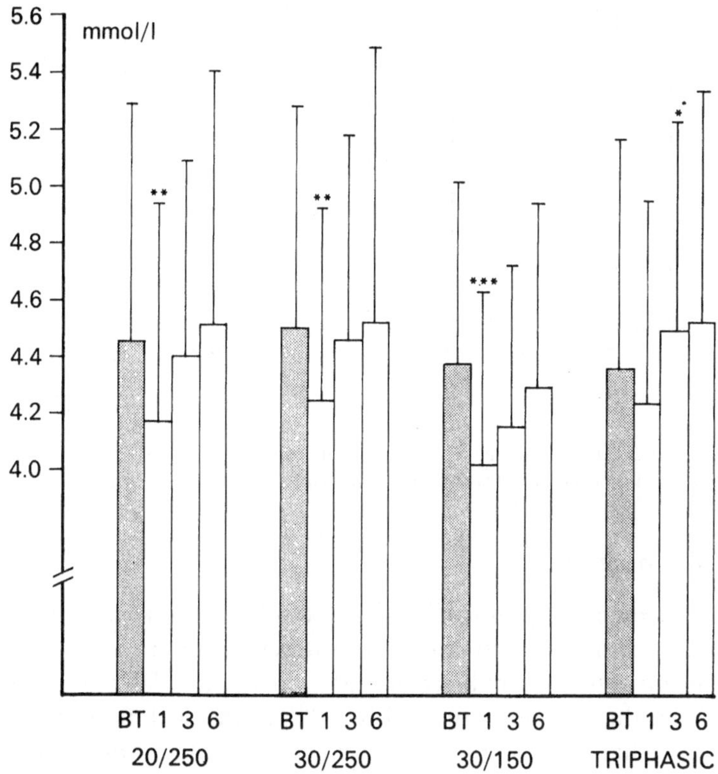

Figure 5.3 The influence of four different combined oral contraceptives on cholesterol concentrations in plasma (mean ± SD). Key as in Figure 5.1

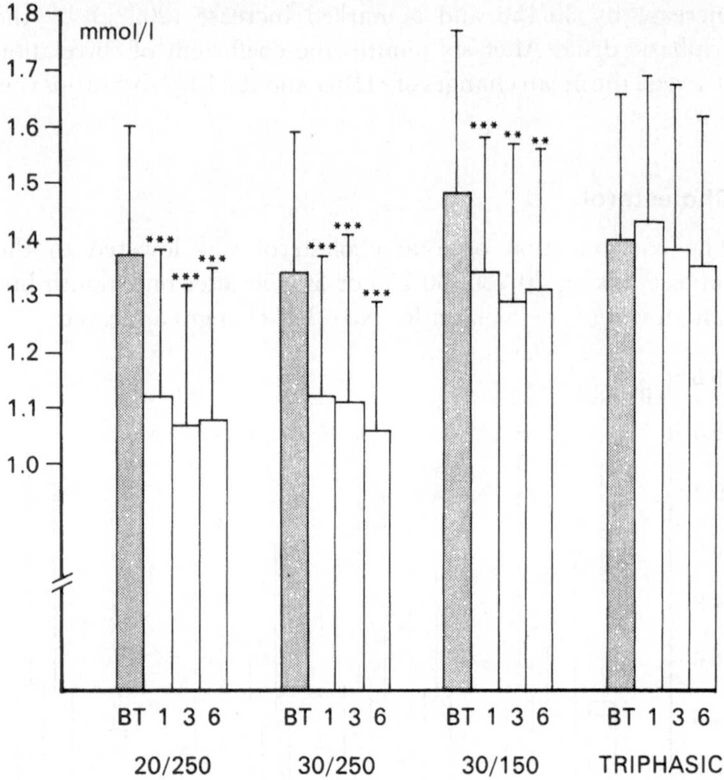

Figure 5.4 The influence of four different combined oral contraceptives on HDL-cholesterol concentrations in plasma (mean ± SD). Key as in Figure 5.1

HDL-cholesterol

In all treatment groups HDL-cholesterol reached a stable level already during the first month of treatment. After six months the concentration was reduced by 20% in the 20/250 group, by 18% in the 30/250 group and by 10% in the 30/150 group. It was unchanged among those taking the triphasic drug. The coefficient of correlation between the mean percentage changes of the HDL-cholesterol and the EE/LNg ratios of the four groups was 0.979. The coefficient of correlation between the mean percentage changes of the HDL-cholesterol and the percentage changes of SHBG of the four groups was 0.915.

HDL-cholesterol: total cholesterol ratio

Table 5.2 shows the means of the HDL-cholesterol: total cholesterol ratio in all groups and at all sampling intervals. 20/250 and 30/250 reduced the HDL-cholesterol: total cholesterol ratio significantly already during the first month of treatment while 30/150 and the triphasic drug had much less influence on this important parameter.

Phospholipids

The mean concentration of total phospholipids was unchanged in three of the groups but was raised in the triphasic group after three and six months.

HDL-phospholipids

The changes were parallel to those of HDL-cholesterol although they were less marked. After six months the coefficient of correlation between the mean percentage changes of the HDL-phospholipids and the EE/LNg ratios of the four groups was 0.996.

Table 5.2 Effects of the four drugs on the HDL-cholesterol: total cholesterol ratio

Drug	*Months of treatment*			
	0	*1*	*3*	*6*
20/250	0.32	0.28†	0.25†	0.25†
30/250	0.30	0.27†	0.26†	0.24†
30/150	0.35	0.34	0.32*	0.32*
Triphasic	0.33	0.34	0.31	0.31*

* = $p < 0.05$ † = $p < 0.001$

Triglycerides

The mean triglyceride levels increased in all groups. After three months the rise was 8% in the 20/250 group, 16% in the 30/250 group, 14% in the 30/150 group and 30% in the triphasic group. At this time interval the coefficient of correlation between the mean percentage changes of the triglyceride levels and the EE/LNg ratios of the four groups was 0.949. After six months the coefficient was reduced to 0.629 due to an unexplained increase in the 20/250 group.

DISCUSSION

Oestrogens raise the plasma triglyceride levels while progestagens of the 19-nortestosterone type seem to be anti-oestrogenic in this respect[3]. A previous study from this laboratory[4] suggested that oestrogens also raise the HDL-cholesterol and that levonorgestrel has an opposite effect. The present results confirm this observation.

The finding that there were linear relations between the EE/LNg ratios and the HDL-cholesterol, HDL-phospholipids and SHBG is interesting. It seems to confirm that SHBG may be used in order to determine the oestrogenity of an oral contraceptive drug. It also shows that HDL levels increase if the drug is highly oestrogenic and are reduced if the gestagenic component dominates. A similar pattern seems to exist also for the triglyceride levels. It is however highly likely that a relation of this type is valid only within a fairly limited dose range.

It can be concluded that of the different EE/LNg combinations investigated the 30/150 and the triphasic drug had least negative effects on the HDL-lipids. The rise of the triglyceride levels which was most prominent with the triphasic drug is also noteworthy even if it was moderate and the treatment levels were within the normal range. 20/250 and 30/250 however induced changes of the HDL-cholesterol: total cholesterol ratio that must be considered as highly unwanted, at least if they are prescribed for a longer period of time.

References

1. Gordon, T., Castelli, W. P., Hjortland, M. C. and Kannel, W. B. (1977). The prediction of coronary heart disease by high-density and other lipoproteins: an historical perspective. In Rifkind, B. M. and Levy, R. I., (eds.) *Hyperlipidemia*, p. 71. (New York: Grune and Stratton)
2. Steinberg, D. (1978). The rediscovery of high density lipoprotein: a negative risk factor in atherosclerosis. *Eur. J. Clin. Invest.*, **8**, 107
3. Larsson-Cohn, U., Berlin, R. and Vikrot, O. (1970). Effects of combined and low dose gestagen oral contraceptives on plasma lipids including individual phospholipids. *Acta Endocrinol. (Kbh.)*, **63**, 717
4. Larsson-Cohn, U., Wallentin, L. and Zador, G. (1979). Plasma lipids and high density lipoproteins during oral contraception with different combinations of ethinyl estradiol and levonorgestrel. *Horm. Metab. Res.*, **11**, 437

6
A randomized study of metabolic effects of four oral contraceptive preparations containing levonorgestrel plus ethinyloestradiol in different regimens

M. BRIGGS and M. BRIGGS

ABSTRACT

Healthy, normotensive, well-motivated, young women were assigned at random to one of four oral contraceptives containing levonorgestrel plus ethinyloestradiol (21-day cyclic treatments) and 80 completed six treatment cycles. Metabolic and endocrine status tests were conducted in the pretreatment cycle and at intervals during the study. All four products appeared to be equally efficient inhibitors of ovulation, as judged by plasma hormone indices. Deterioration of oral glucose tolerance and insulin responses were noted with all preparations, except a triphasic formulation. All products increased the concentration of triglycerides in fasting plasma, though the extent of the increase appeared to be dose-related. Only the highest dose product significantly increased plasma cholesterol. Cholesterol in high-density lipoproteins was significantly increased by an oestrogenic biphasic product, but significantly decreased by a high-dose fixed combination. Significant increases in fibrinogen, plasminogen, and coagulation factors VII, VIII and X were observed, especially with the highest dose product and the oestrogen-dominated biphasic. Antithrombin III was suppressed. Renin activity and renin-substrate concentration were elevated, while plasma renin concentration was reduced: again the effects appeared to be related to the oestrogen dose.

INTRODUCTION

Since their introduction more than a generation ago, the use of oral contraceptives containing combinations of a synthetic oestrogen and synthetic progestagen[1] have proved the most effective method of family planning[2]. Indeed, of contraceptive methods they rank only second to surgical sterilization. A large epidemiological investigation[3] has suggested that oral contraceptive users may have an increased risk of mortality when compared to non-users (who may be using other contraceptive methods), while a smaller investigation[4] has found increased mortality as compared to users of other methods. Both investigations suggest that oral contraceptives protect to some extent against neoplastic disease, but increase cardiovascular risks. The situation is complicated by a positive association between oral contraceptive use and other cardiovascular risk factors, especially cigarette smoking[5]. Studies of cardiovascular mortality in young women in a variety of countries have failed to find any evidence for an effect of oral contraceptive use[6], while a reanalysis[7] of available risk factors has found that mortality in non-smoking oral contraceptive users is less than that of non-users, or users of barrier contraceptive methods, up to the age of 40 years.

Despite this controversy, there is widespread concern to

reduce potential cardiovascular risks in oral contraceptive users. Differences between formulations for effects on laboratory parameters of cardiovascular risk (lipids, coagulation factors, altered blood pressure) have been proposed as a basis for selecting particular oral contraceptives for general use[8].

Commercially available oral contraceptive steroids present little choice. Mestranol is extensively metabolized to ethinyloestradiol by the human liver, and the two are bioequivalent over the usual contraceptive dose range[9]. Of the many available progestagens, 17α-acetoxyprogestagens (such as megestrol acetate, chlormadinone acetate, medroxyprogesterone acetate etc.) have been withdrawn in many countries (wrongly in the view of the present authors) on the results of chronic toxicity in dogs[10]. Compounds in the norethisterone series (ethynodiol diacetate, lynestrenol, norethisterone acetate, etc.) are metabolically and, probably, biologically equivalent[11]. Of the totally synthetic gonanes, norgestrel is a mixture of two enantiomers of which levonorgestrel is the hormonally active form[12]. Other gonanes, such as norgestimate (the 3-oxime of levonorgestrel-17-acetate) and ORG 2969 (3-deoxy-11-methylenelevonorgestrel), are metabolized to levonorgestrel, or closely related compounds[13,14], and clinical experience with them is very limited.

As levonorgestrel can be used clinically at a significantly lower dose than norethisterone, is not associated with a number of biochemical changes seen with norethisterone, has higher affinity for the plasma carrier-protein (so that the plasma free pool size is reduced), and has significant antagonistic effects on potentially adverse oestrogen-medicated metabolic changes, it is the progestagen to be preferred[15,16].

A number of combinations of levonorgestrel (LNg) with ethinyloestradiol (EE) are available in various countries. These vary considerably in overall dosage and oestrogen:progestagen ratio. The present study was conducted to compare metabolic effects of four different formulations under carefully controlled conditions.

METHODS AND MATERIALS

Using random number tables, healthy young women were assigned to one of the four different oral contraceptive formulations under test. The women were informed of the nature of the study and provided informed consent. All were seeking reliable oral contraception for family planning. None had used any form of hormonal contraception for at least six cycles prior to beginning treatment. Other criteria for entering the study included a complete personal and family history with no absolute or relative contraindications to oral contraceptives[17], regular cycles, a body weight within 10% of the ideal for body height, no concurrent medications, normotension, and good personal motivation. The majority were nurses or postgraduate students. Age range was 19 to 30 years (mean 24 ± 2.5).

Table 6.1 Oral contraceptive formulations

No.	*Code*	*Regimen (days)*	*Composition*
1.	250/50	21	250 μg levonorgestrel + 50 μg ethinyloestradiol
2.	150/30	21	150 μg levonorgestrel + 30 μg ethinyloestradiol
3.	Biphasic*	10	50 μg levonorgestrel + 50 μg ethinyloestradiol
		11	125 μg levonorgestrel + 50 μg ethinyloestradiol
4.	Triphasic	6	50 μg levonorgestrel + 30 μg ethinyloestradiol
		5	75 μg levonorgestrel + 40 μg ethinyloestradiol
		10	125 μg levonorgestrel + 30 μg ethinyloestradiol

* Sometimes used with seven placebos in the treatment-free interval

During the immediate pretreatment cycle the volunteers were advised to use a barrier method of contraception. All oral contraceptives were started on cycle day 5 of the first treatment cycle. There were 21 doses per cycle, followed by a 7-day treatment-free interval (a small number of subjects received placebo tablets during this interval).

All subjects were required to provide one fasting blood

specimen during the pretreatment cycle (taken as part of an oral glucose tolerance test) and further specimens during the late stage of subsequent cycles.

Composition of the four oral contraceptive preparations used is set out in Table 6.1. All were commercial products supplied by either Schering A.G. (Berlin) or Wyeth International Limited (Philadelphia).

References to laboratory methods are set out in Table 6.2.

Table 6.2 Laboratory methods

Parameter	*Reference*
Progesterone	Johansson (1970)[18]
Oestradiol	Edqvist and Johansson (1972)[19]
Luteinizing hormone (LH)	Karonen *et al.* (1978)[20]
Follicle-stimulating hormone (FSH)	Karonen *et al.* (1978)[20]
Glucose	Cramp (1967)[21]
Insulin	Herbert *et al.* (1965)[22]
Cholesterol	Robertson and Cramp (1970)[31]
Triglycerides	Cramp and Robertson (1968)[32]
High-density lipoprotein (HDL)-cholesterol	Burstein and Samaille (1960)[33]
Fibrinogen	Clauss (1957)[23]
Factor VII	Poller *et al.* (1971)[24]
Factor VIII	Breckenridge and Ratnoff (1962)[25]
Factor X	Aurell *et al.* (1978)[26]
Antithrombin III	Abllgaard *et al.* (1976)[27]
Plasminogen	Soria *et al.* (1975)[28]
Renin activity	Delorme *et al.* (1976)[29]
Renin-substrate concentration	Campillo *et al.* (1976)[30]
Renin concentration	Campillo *et al.* (1976)[30]

RESULTS

Endocrine indices of ovulation

Small numbers of women from each treatment group volunteered to provide blood specimens for 7 consecutive days during the middle of their pretreatment cycle, then again during

Table 6.3 Mean peak concentrations of plasma gonadotropins

Product	*Number of women*	*Plasma gonadotropins Main peak concentrations (sampled on days 11, 12, 13, 14, 15, 16, 17) (IU/l)*			
		*LH**		*FSH†*	
		Pretreatment	*Cycle 1*	*Pretreatment*	*Cycle 1*
250/50	5	105 ± 19	13 ± 6	12.5 ± 3.1	4.8 ± 1.9
150/30	6	109 ± 11	17 ± 8	13.6 ± 3.4	5.0 ± 1.6
Biphasic	4	98 ± 13	19 ± 6	11.9 ± 3.8	4.5 ± 2.1
Triphasic	7	115 ± 16	12 ± 5	13.8 ± 2.9	4.9 ± 1.4

*Second IRP–hMG standard
†NIH–FSH–S1 standard

treatment cycle 1. Specimens were collected on cycle days 11 to 17 and were analysed for LH and FSH. The maximum concentrations of each hormone in the two series of blood specimens were selected. Table 6.3 shows that the mean maxima in the pretreatment cycle ranged from 98 to 115 IU/l for LH, and from 11.9 to 13.8 IU/l for FSH. In contrast, during treatment cycle 1 mean maxima for LH were 12 to 19 IU/l, and for FSH were 4.5 to 5.0 IU/l.

Examination of individual results revealed that all 22 women included in this part of the study showed midcycle gonadotropin plasma surges, but these were absent during the use of any of the oral contraceptives.

Plasma concentrations of oestradiol were measured in these same women for blood specimens collected on days 13 and 14 of their pretreatment, first and third cycles. Additional specimens taken on days 22 and 23 were analysed for plasma progesterone. A few additional women who were unable to take part in the gonadotropin study also supplied blood on days 13, 14, 22 and 23 of their pretreatment and third cycles.

Mean results for these two hormones are shown in Table 6.4. Midcycle plasma oestradiol ranged from 1.10 to 1.28 nmol/l pretreatment, but fell to 0.15 to 0.21 nmol/l during cycle 3 (the smaller number of cycle 1 results were not significantly different to those seen in cycle 3). Similarly, the late cycle plasma progesterone concentrations ranged from 25.2 to 31.9 nmol/l pretreatment, but were only 1.8 to 2.0 nmol/l during cycle 3 (cycle 1 results were similarly low).

Table 6.4 Endogenous sex hormone concentrations in plasma*

OC product	*Cycle*	*Number of women*	*Mean hormone concentrations ± SD (nmol/l)*	
			Oestradiol (days 13 and 14)	*Progesterone (days 22 and 23)*
250 μg LNg + 50 μg EE	0	6	1.28 ± 0.29	25.2 ± 3.6
	3	6	0.15 ± 0.08	1.8 ± 0.70
150 μg LNg + 30 μg EE	0	8	1.10 ± 0.27	31.9 ± 3.8
	3	8	0.21 ± 0.09	2.0 ± 0.58
Biphasic†	0	9	1.18 ± 0.23	27.1 ± 2.9
	3	9	0.18 ± 0.06	1.6 ± 0.51
Triphasic‡	0	7	1.13 ± 0.31	31.3 ± 3.7
	3	7	0.20 ± 0.07	1.9 ± 0.62

* Measured by RIA (differences between products in cycle 0 are statistically insignificant: for each product (both hormones) differences between cycles 0 and 3 are significant at $p<0.05$)
† 50 μg LNg + 50 μg EE (× 11); 125 μg LNg + 50 μg EE (× 10)
‡ 50 μg LNg + 30 μg EE (× 6); 75 μg LNg + 40 μg EE (× 5); 125 μg LNg + 30 μg EE (× 10)

Glucose tolerance

Results of oral glucose tolerance tests (1 g/kg), together with plasma immunoreactive insulin responses, are shown in Figure 6.1. The mean values for each group are presented pretreatment, then during the sixth treatment cycle (days 20 to 25). Statistically significant deterioration of glucose response curves occurred with the highest dose product (250 μg LNg + 50 μg EE) and with the biphasic preparation (see Table 6.1). No significant differences in glucose tolerance curves were seen with the lower dose combination (150 μg LNg + 30 μg EE) or with

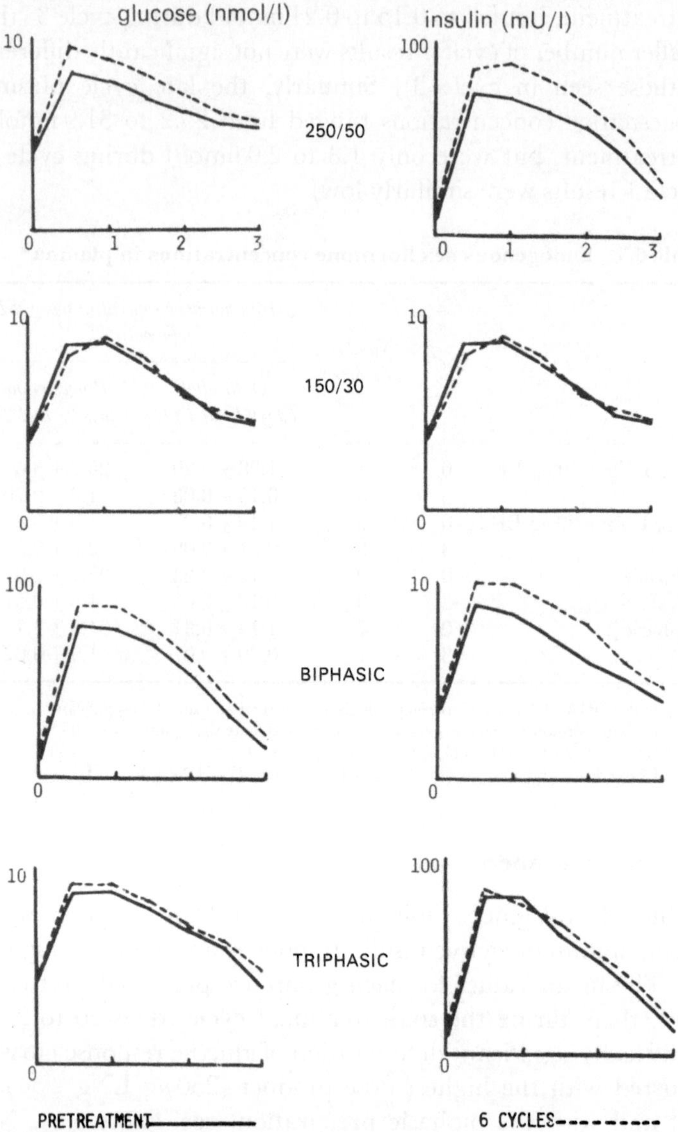

Figure 6.1 Results of oral glucose tolerance tests (1 g/kg), with plasma immunoreactive insulin responses

the triphasic preparation (see Table 6.1). In contrast, plasma insulin responses during the glucose tolerance tests were significantly higher at 6 months than pretreatment for all products except the triphasic preparation.

Plasma lipids

Each woman in the study provided a blood specimen each cycle (days 22–25) after an overnight fast (checked by blood glucose). Mean lipid values for the four treatment groups over 6 cycles are shown in Figure 6.2. Each individual woman's results in the three tests (HDL-cholesterol, total cholesterol, triglycerides) during the pretreatment cycle were taken as 100 and values in subsequent tests were recalculated on this basis.

As compared to the pretreatment values, HDL-cholesterol concentration was significantly ($p<0.05$) depressed by the highest dose product (250 μg LNg + 50 μg EE), but significantly elevated by the biphasic preparation. The changes seen with 150 μg LNg + 30 μg EE or the triphasic preparation were not statistically significant.

For plasma total cholesterol, the only oral contraceptive product to induce a statistically significant change at 6 cycles was 250 μg LNg + 50 μg EE, though the mean change was small (+5%). In contrast, this product, and also the biphasic preparation, were associated with a large increase in fasting plasma triglycerides (*circa* 30%). The increase in plasma triglycerides seen with the triphasic preparation was much less (+16%), but was also statistically significant, though the change (+6%) seen with 150 μg LNg + 30 μg EE was not.

Coagulation and fibrinolytic factors

Figures 6.3A and 6.3B present the changes in these factors associated with the four oral contraceptive products. Measurements were made on blood specimens collected during cycles 0,

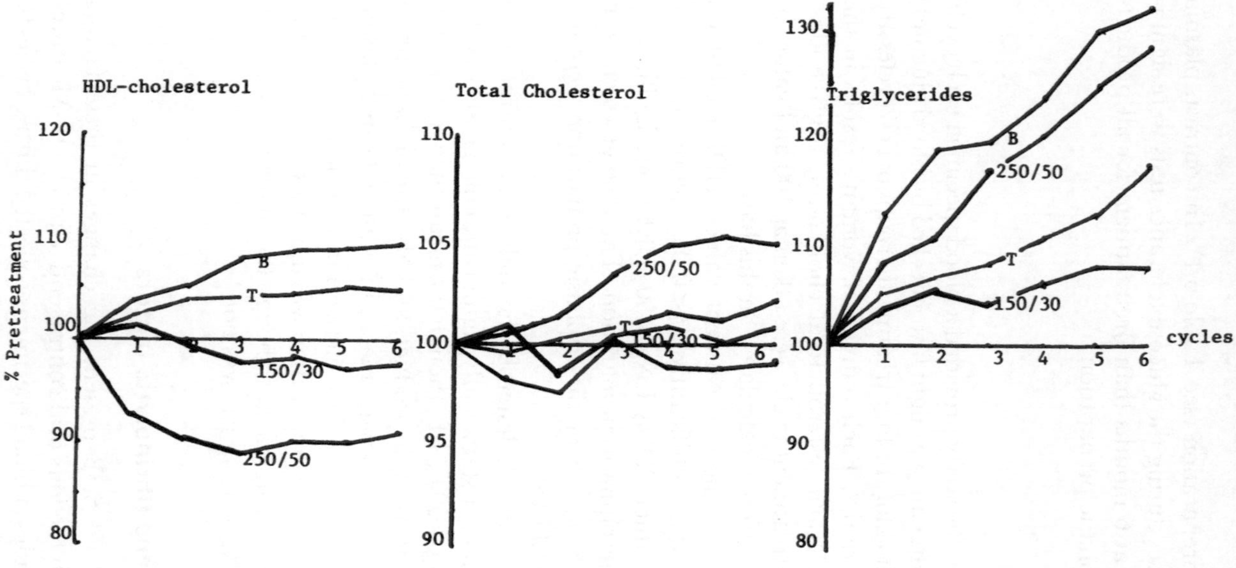

Figure 6.2 Changes in fasting plasma lipids in 80 young women assigned at random to four different combined OC. Key: B = Biphasic preparation (see Table 6.1); T = Triphasic preparation (see Table 6.1); 150/30 = 150 μg LNg + 30 μg EE; 250/50 = 250 μg LNg + 50 μg EE

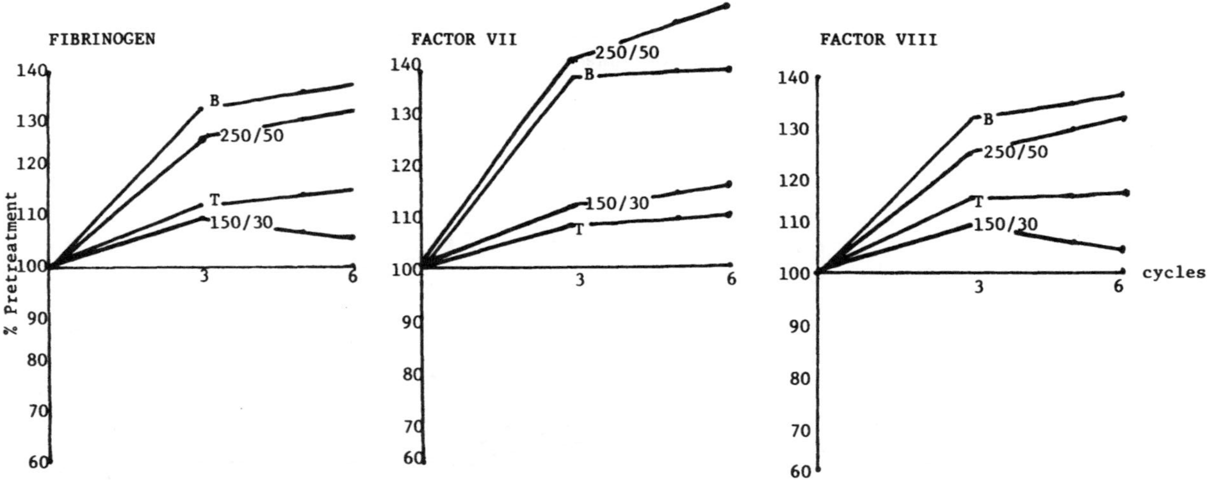

Figure 6.3A Changes in blood coagulation factors and related parameters in 80 young women assigned at random to four different combined OC. Key as Figure 6.2

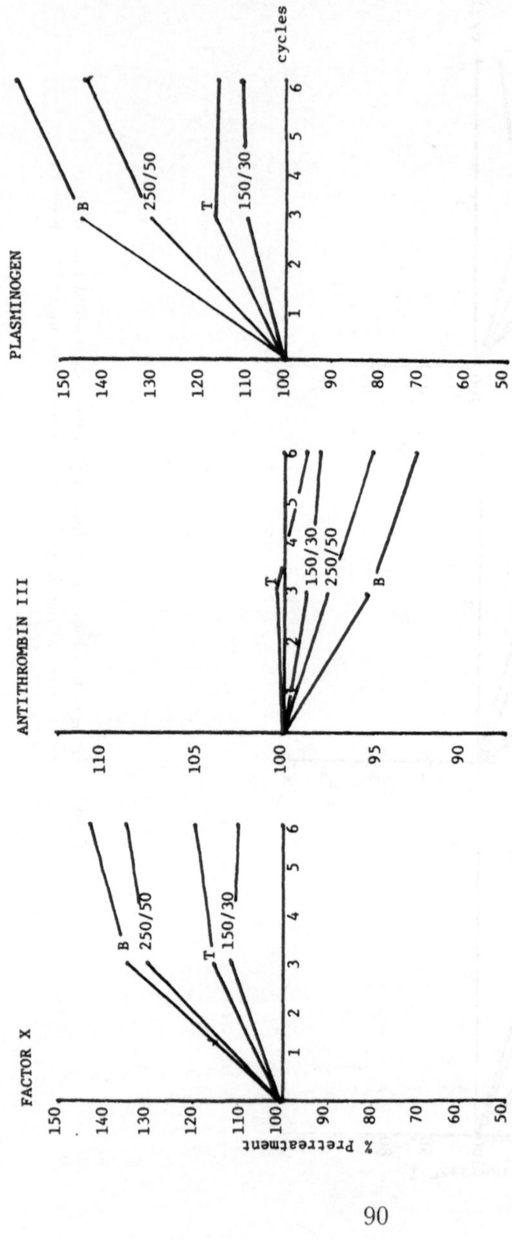

Figure 6.3B Changes in blood coagulation factors and related parameters in 80 young women assigned at random to four different combined OC. Key as Figure 6.2

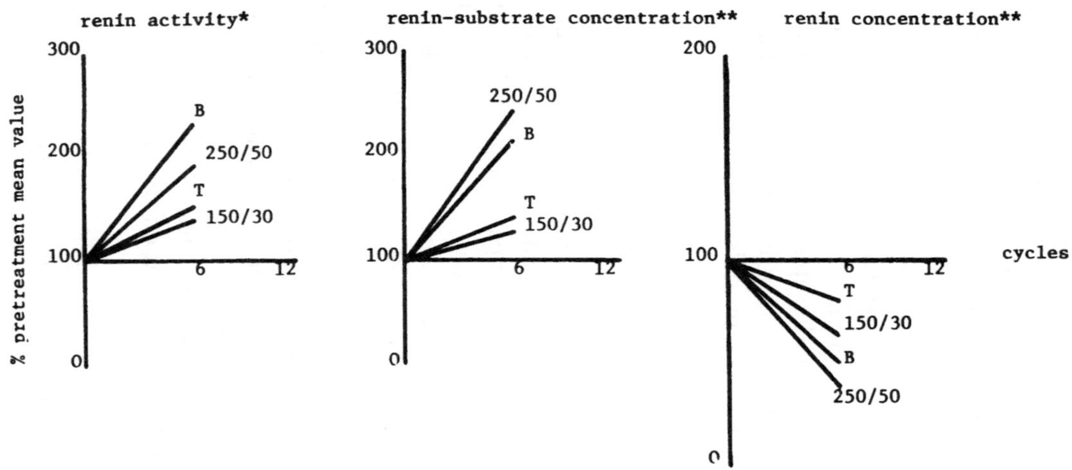

Figure 6.4 Changes in plasma renin–angiotensin system. * angiotensin-I formed after incubation of dialysed plasma at 37 °C; ** angiotensin-I formed after incubation of plasma with excess added renin; *** angiotensin-I formed after incubation of plasma with excess added renin-substrate. Products are as in Figures 6.2 and 6.3 (80 normotensive women randomized)

3, and 6. It will be seen that large changes occurred with many factors, but that most changes occurred by cycle 3 and subsequent further alterations were generally much smaller.

Again the pretreatment result for each factor was taken as 100 and later determinations recalculated on that basis.

The two most oestrogenic preparations (250 μg LNg + 50 μg EE and the biphasic) were associated with a highly significant ($p < 0.001$) increase in fibrinogen, factors VII, VIII, X, and plasminogen. Both also significantly suppressed antithrombin-III. Changes with 150 μg LNg + 30 μg EE and the triphasic preparation were much less, usually only 10 to 15% of pretreatment values.

Renin–angiotensin system

No woman in this study became hypertensive (blood pressure higher than 140/90 mmHg) during treatment, despite large changes in their renin–angiotensin systems. Several showed small (*c.* 5 to 10 mmHg) increases in reported systolic and diastolic pressures, but such changes are most difficult to quantify without a strict clinical protocol specifically designed to detect such small changes.

Blood was collected from supine subjects for investigations of renin activity, renin-substrate concentration, and renin concentration during cycles 0 and 6. A further measurement will be made during cycle 12.

Again pretreatment values for the three tests have been taken as 100 and subsequent results calculated on this basis (Figure 6.4).

With the two highest oestrogen dose products (250 μg LNg + 50 μg EE and the biphasic), renin activity and renin-substrate concentration approximately doubled ($p < 0.001$). In contrast, renin concentration was reduced to around 30 to 40% of pretreatment values ($p < 0.001$) with these two products.

Changes with the two lower dose products were less, but still statistically significant ($p < 0.01$). The increase in renin activity was 20 to 30%, in renin-substrate concentration 12 to 20%, while the fall in renin concentration was about 15 to 20%.

DISCUSSION AND CONCLUSIONS

During the 480 treatment cycles with the four different products there were no pregnancies. Although the number of women examined was small, all four oral contraceptives appeared to be good, and equally effective, inhibitors of ovulation, as judged from the midcycle suppression of plasma gonadotropins and oestradiol concentrations, and the absence of a late cycle rise in plasma progesterone level. This inhibition occurred during the first treatment cycle.

As has been previously reported many times[34,35], many oral contraceptives induce significant alterations in glucose tolerance tests and plasma insulin responses. Both oestrogen and progestagen components may be implicated in this effect. It is of interest that in the present study the two lower dose formulations did not significantly alter glucose tolerance, while the triphasic preparation had no effect on insulin responses.

It is widely accepted (see reviews by Briggs *et al.*[34], Briggs[35]) that large increases in fasting plasma triglycerides, accompanied by small increases in cholesterol, occur during oral contraception. At 6 cycles, the increases with the biphasic preparation and 250 μg LNg + 50 μg EE were statistically indistinguishable. The lowest fixed-dose combination (150 μg LNg + 30 μg EE) produced a statistically insignificant small increase, while the rise with the triphasic preparation was intermediate.

The drop in HDL-cholesterol, accompanied by the increase in total cholesterol, seen with 250 μg LNg + 50 μg EE suggests a large increase in the β-lipoprotein fractions. The overall changes increase atherogenic risks. In contrast, the other three products do not significantly alter total cholesterol, though the biphasic preparation increases HDL-cholesterol (and presumably reduces β-lipoprotein cholesterol).

Changes in coagulation and fibrinolytic factors were similar for 250 μg LNg + 50 μg EE and the biphasic preparation. They were generally dramatic. In contrast, the triphasic preparation and 150 μg LNg + 30 μg EE produced similar, and much smaller, changes.

While there is no generally agreed laboratory test for a hypercoagulable state, prudence would support the use of products which induce the smallest possible alterations in the delicate and complicated systems regulating human blood coagulation.

Finally, changes induced by oral contraceptives in the renin–angiotensin system are also spectacular. The mechanism is probably an oestrogen-mediated stimulation of hepatic secretion of the renin-substrates (several closely related proteins called angiotensinogens). These are acted upon by renins and other peptidases to release angiotensin I, II and III, which have direct hypertensive effects on arterioles, as well as triggering release of aldosterone.

Again the two high oestrogen formulations produce similar, and statistically indistinguishable, increases in plasma concentration of renin-substrate. The two lower dose products have much less effect. The other observed changes follow from this increase. Renin activity increases approximately in proportion to the substrate concentration, while renin concentration is reduced by the operation of a feedback mechanism on renin release.

In selecting an oral contraceptive a number of interrelated factors need to be considered. First, the formulation must approach 100% effectiveness when properly used. Secondly, the incidence of menstrual irregularities must be acceptable to the user. Finally, the effect of the product on laboratory risk indicators must be minimal. Most oestrogen–progestagen combinations show similar high efficacy as oral contraceptives[1], though that of progestagen minipills is significantly less. The latter products also lead to significant menstrual irregularities[36]. Reducing the dose of fixed-dose combinations also retains efficacy, but again may lead to problems of menstrual irregularity, at least in the first few treatment cycles[37,38].

With particular reference to the four products compared in the present study, all appear to be equally effective contraceptives. Good cycle control is given by 250 μg LNg + 50 μg EE[37,39], the biphasic[40,41], and triphasic[42,43] formulations. The lower fixed-dose preparation (150 μg LNg + 30 μg EE) provides initially less acceptable cycle control than the others[44–46].

In terms of metabolic effects, the choice seems clear. Both 250 μg LNg + 50 μg EE and the biphasic preparation significantly alter glucose tolerance, insulin response, plasma lipids, coagulation/fibrinolytic factors, and the renin–angiotensin system. The other two products have either no effect, or much less impact, on these biochemical parameters. Either 150 μg LNg + 30 μg EE or the triphasic preparation would be a logical first choice, but if initial menstrual irregularities are likely to be a problem, the triphasic becomes the product to be selected for most women starting oral contraception.

References

1. Briggs, M. H. (1977a). Combined oral contraceptives. In *Regulation of Human Fertility*, pp. 253–282. (Copenhagen: Scriptor)
2. Hawkins, D. F. and Elder, M. G. (1979). *Human Fertility Control*, pp. 49–91. (London: Butterworths)
3. Berel, V. and Kay, C. R. (1977). Mortality among oral contraceptive users. *Lancet*, **2**, 727
4. Vessey, M. P., McPherson, K. and Johnson, B. (1977). Mortality among women participating in the Oxford/Family Planning Association Contraceptive Study. *Lancet*, **2**, 731
5. Royal College of General Practitioners (1974). *Oral Contraceptives and Health*, pp. 10–11. (London: Pitman)
6. Belsey, M. A., Russell, Y. and Kinnear, K. (1979). Cardiovascular disease and oral contraceptives: a reappraisal of vital statistics data. *Fam. Plann. Perspect.*, **11**, 84

7. Tieze, C. (1979). The pill and mortality from cardiovascular disease: another look. *Fam. Plann. Perspect.*, **11**, 80
8. Briggs, M. H. (1979a). Recent biological studies in relation to low dose hormonal contraceptives. *Br. J. Fam. Plann.*, **5**, 25
9. Goldzieher, J. W., De La Pena, A., Chenault, C. B. and Cervantes, A. (1975). Comparative studies of the ethynyl estrogens used in oral contraceptives. *Am. J. Obstet. Gynecol.*, **122**, 615, 619, 625
10. Briggs, M. H. (1977b). The beagle dog and contraceptive steroids. *Life Sci.*, **21**, 275
11. Fortherby, K. and James, F. (1972). Metabolism of synthetic steroids. *Adv. Ster. Biochem. Pharmacol.*, **3**, 67
12. Jones, R. C., Singer, A. C. and Edgren, R. A. (1979). The biological activities of norgestrel and its enantiomers. *Int. J. Fertil.*, **24**, 39
13. Sisenwine, S. F., Liu, A. L., Kimmel, H. B. and Ruelius, H. W. (1977). Conversion of *d*-norgestrel-3-oxime-17-acetate to *d*-norgestrel in female rhesus monkeys. *Contraception*, **15**, 27
14. Viinikka, L., Ylikorkala, O., Vihko, B., Wijnaad, H. P. and Booij, M. (1979). Metabolism of a new synthetic progestogen, ORG 2969, in female volunteers. *Eur. J. Clin. Pharmacol.*, **15**, 349
15. Briggs, M. H. and Briggs, M. (1976). Molecular biology and oral contraception. *N.Z. Med. J.*, **83**, 257
16. Briggs, M. H. (1979b). Biochemical basis for the selection of oral contraceptives. *Int. J. Gynaecol. Obstet.*, **16**, 509
17. Briggs, M. H. and Briggs, M. (1980). Relative contraindications to oral contraceptives and their use in adolescence, puerperium, and menopause. *Proceedings of the 4th International Meeting on Fertility Control*, Genoa, in press. (Palermo: Cofese Edizioni)
18. Johansson, E. D. B. (1970). Simplified procedure for the assay of progesterone. *Acta Endocrinol. Suppl.*, **147**, 188
19. Edqvist, L. E. and Johansson, E. D. B. (1972). Radioimmunoassay of oestrone and oestradiol in human and bovine peripheral plasma. *Acta Endocrinol.*, **71**, 716
20. Karonen, S. L., Lähteenmäki, P., Hohenthal, U., Aldercreutz, H. (1978). Evaluation of the double antibody–solid phase radioimmunoassay technique in plasma LH and FSH. *Scand. J. Clin. Invest.*, **38**, 1
21. Cramp, D. G. (1967). New automated enzymatic method for measuring glucose by glucose oxidase. *J. Clin. Pathol.*, **20**, 910
22. Herbert, V., Lau, K., Gottleib, C. W., Bleicher, S. J. (1965). Coated charcoal immunoassay of insulin. *J. Clin. Endocrinol. Metab.*, **25**, 1375
23. Clauss, A. (1957). Gerinnungsphysiologische Schnellmethode zur Bastimmuny des Fibrinogens. *Acta Haematol.*, **17**, 237
24. Poller, L., Thomson, J. M., Sear, C. H. J., Thomas, W. (1971). Identification of a congenital defect of factor VII in a colony of beagle dogs: clinical use of the plasma. *J. Clin. Pathol.*, **24**, 626
25. Breckenridge, R. T. and Ratnoff, O. D. (1962). Studies on the nature of

the circulating anticoagulant directed against antihaemophilic factors. *Blood*, **20**, 137

26. Aurell, L., Simonsson, R., Arielly, S., Karlsson, G., Friberger, P., Claesan, G. (1978). Chromogenic peptide substrates for factor Xa. *Haemostasis*, **7**, 92
27. Abllgaard, U., Lie, M., Odegard, O. R. (1976). Antithrombin assay with new chromogenic substrates (S-2238 and Chromozym TH). *Thromb. Res.*, **11**, 549
28. Soria, J., Soria, C., Samama, M. (1975). Measurement of plasminogen using chromogenic tripeptide. *Organization des Laboratorires-Biologie Prospective III' Collegue de point-a-moussan. L/Expansion Scientifique Française*
29. Delorme, A., Guyene, P. T., Corvol, P., Menard, J. (1976). Methodologic problems in plasma renin activity measurements. *Am. J. Med.*, **61**, 725
30. Campillo, J. E., Del Rio, C. G., Quesada, T., Osorio, C. (1976). Simultaneous measurement of renin and renin substrate concentration in human plasma by a simple kinetic method. *Clin. Chim. Acta*, **73**, 475
31. Robertson, G. and Cramp, D. G. (1970). Evaluation of cholesterol determination in serum and serum lipoprotein fractions by semi-automated fluorimetric method. *J. Clin. Pathol.*, **23**, 243
32. Cramp, D. G. and Robertson, G. (1968). Fluorimetric assay of triglycerides by a semi-automated method. *Anal. Biochem.*, **25**, 246
33. Burstein, M. and Samaille, J. (1960). Rapid method for cholesterol in serum α and β lipoproteins. *Clin. Chim. Acta*, **5**, 609
34. Briggs, M. H., Pitchford, A. G., Staniford, M., Barker, H. M. and Taylor, D. (1970). Metabolic effects of steroid contraceptives. *Adv. Steroid Biochem. Pharmacol.*, **2**, 111
35. Briggs, M. (1975). Biochemical effects of oral contraceptives. *Adv. Steroid Biochem. Pharmacol.*, **5**, 65
36. Fotherby, K. (1977). Low doses of gestagens as fertility regulating agents. In Diczfalusy, E. (ed.) *Regulation of Human Fertility*, pp. 283–322. Copenhagen: Scriptor
37. Briggs, M. and Briggs, M. H. (1977). Low dose oral contraceptives. *OB/GYN Digest*, February, 12–16
38. Rozenbaum, H. (1978). Low dose estrogen/progestogen combinations. *Rév. Méd. (Paris)*, **19**, 1821
39. Korba, V. D. and Heil, C. G. (1975). Eight years of fertility control with norgestrel-ethinyl estradiol: an updated clinical review. *Fertil. Steril.*, **26**, 973
40. Larranaga, A., Sartoretto, J. N., Winterhalter, M., Filho, F. N. (1978). Clinical evaluation of two biphasic and one triphasic norgestrel/ethinyl estradiol regimens. *Int. J. Fertil.*, **23**, 193
41. Briggs, M. H. and Briggs (1977). Clinical and biochemical investigations of a variable-dose combined type oral contraceptive. *Curr. Med. Res. Opin.*, **5**, 212
42. Zador, G. (1979). Fertility regulation using triphasic administration of

ethinyl oestradiol and levonorgestrel in comparison with the 30 plus 150 μg fixed dose regime. *Acta Obstet. Gynecol. Scand., Suppl.*, **88**, 43
43. Lachnit-Fixson, U. (1979). The first three-stage preparation for hormonal contraception. Clinical results. *Münch. Med. Wochenschr.*, **121**, 1421
44. Woutersz, T. B. (1975). Profile of a new low dose combination estrogen and progestogen oral contraceptive: a review of nine clinical studies. *J. Reprod. Med.*, **15**, 87
45. Woutersz, T. B. (1976). Three and one-half years' experience with a lower-dose combination oral contraceptive. *J. Reprod. Med.*, **16**, 338
46. Briggs, M. H. and Briggs, M. (1976). Clinical and biochemical investigations of an ultra low-dose combined type oral contraceptive. *Curr. Med. Res. Opin.*, **3**, 618

7
Clinical investigation with a new triphasic oral contraceptive

U. LACHNIT-FIXSON

The extended clinical trial of the two triphasic preparations SH B 264 AB and SH B 261 AB for contraceptive reliability, cycle control and tolerance was carried out in different countries: Austria, the Netherlands, Peru, Venezuela and West Germany. Both clinics and gynaecologists in private practice participated in the trial.

Generally, women were selected on the basis of their meeting the requirements for the prescription of oral contraceptives in accordance with established medical practice. The participants were allocated to the preparations in a randomized fashion and were instructed to use the oral contraceptive as follows: Intake from the first package was to start on the first day of the cycle. After finishing the first calendar package, an interval of 7 days had to be observed as usual, before starting the next package. Before starting medication, all women were told that the first medication cycle would have a duration of only about 23 to 25 days.

RESULTS OF THE COMPARISON

Test preparation SH B 264 AB was given to 696 women for a

total of 6628 cycles. The version SH B 261 AB was given to 634 women for 6025 cycles.

During the computer evaluation of the period of use of SH B 264 AB, no pregnancies were recorded, despite the fact that medication errors (one or several omission of tablets) were admitted. During medication with SH B 261 AB there was one pregnancy, which had to be evaluated as 'drug failure'.

Both preparations were equally well tolerated, but the incidence of spotting and intermenstrual bleeding episodes was somewhat lower for SH B 264 AB than for SH B 261 AB (see Table 7.1).

Table 7.1 Intermenstrual bleeding rate, calculated in terms of the total number of cycles, in %

	SH B 264 AB	*SH B 261 AB*
Spotting	4.6	5.1
Breakthrough bleeding	2.0	2.5
Spotting and breakthrough bleeding*	1.2	1.3

* Beginning as spotting and only later turning into heavier bleeding

Though the differences between the 2 triphasic versions are not large, it was decided to give preference to the preparation SH B 264 AB. The main reason for our decision was that this preparation, with its markedly lower total oestrogen dose per cycle (0.68 mg as against 0.83 mg ethinyloestradiol in SH B 261 AB), meets the criterion of the lowest possible dose of *both* hormone components more closely than the comparison drug.

The following discussion gives a brief summary of the test data for SH B 264 AB.

Duration of treatment

The medication was used by 594 women (=85.3% of all test persons) for 6 cycles, by 362 women (52%) for 12 cycles, and by

71 women (10.2%) for 18 cycles. As previously pointed out, no pregnancy occurred in 6628 treatment cycles in this study.

Cycle control

Similar to other oral contraceptives the trial preparation exerts a normalizing effect on cycle length, duration and intensity of bleeding, especially in women with previously prolonged and/or profuse bleeding episodes. However, in contrast with many one-phase preparations, there is no tendency towards very short or very scanty bleedings, even on prolonged use.

Failure of withdrawal bleeding to occur was extremely rare. Such a 'pseudoamenorrhoea' occurred only in 27 out of a total of 6628 treatment cycles. Thus the amenorrhoea rate amounts to only 0.4%.

Intermenstrual bleeding

All bleeding episodes were recorded separately for the last cycle before start of the trial and in every treatment cycle. In the 264/261 comparison the low overall rates of spotting and BTB have already been shown (Table 7.1).

As with one-phase preparations, intermenstrual bleeding occurred particularly at the beginning of treatment. With increasing duration of treatment the bleeding rates drop continuously.

Since 1973, in evaluating the test results of various oral contraceptives[1–4], we could show repeatedly that there is a positive correlation between the incidence of spotting and breakthrough bleeding and the omission of tablets. We also noted that women who had a history of intermenstrual bleeding complain more often of these disturbances when taking ovulation inhibitors than women without such a positive history.

These observations also apply to this triphasic preparation.

Table 7.2 shows how important correct intake of medication is for good cycle control. Spotting and especially breakthrough bleeding occur considerably more frequently in cycles with intake errors.

Of all the women in the collective 16.3% had reported intermenstrual bleeding episodes in their history; 7.5% of all women in the control cycle immediately before the beginning of medication had intermenstrual bleeding.

Table 7.2 Intermenstrual bleeding under SH B 264 AB in 6547 cycles

	Without errors in tablet-taking (6341 cycles)	*With errors in tablet-taking* (116 cycles)*
Spotting	4.5%	11.2%
Breakthrough bleeding	1.8%	13.8%
Spotting and breakthrough bleeding†	1.2%	1.7%

* Error in tablet-taking = tablets forgotten
† Beginning as spotting and only later turning into heavier bleeding

The separate evaluation of women with and without bleeding abnormalities of this kind again confirmed with this triphasic preparation that a history of bleeding plays a major role. Thus, for example, the spotting rate in women with such a history was 18.9% in the first medication cycle, whereas in women without a positive history the spotting rate was only 8.1%.

For this reason the group of women without a history of intermenstrual bleeding episodes and without medication errors is the most suitable for recognizing disturbances that can truly be traced to the test preparation. On the basis of 5273 SH B 264 AB cycles without a medication error in women without a history of intermenstrual bleeding, the rates of intermenstrual bleeding were very low: spotting in 3.7% of cycles, breakthrough bleeding in 1.5% of cycles, and spotting and breakthrough bleeding in 1.3% of cycles.

Tolerance and side-effects

In the vast majority of women body weight and blood pressure values remained practically constant. In no case was it necessary to discontinue medication prematurely because of a rise in blood pressure.

The following side-effects were recorded as subjective: dysmenorrhoea, nausea and vomiting, dizziness, breast tension, headaches, nervousness and changes in libido. Indications about these symptoms were recorded in the last cycle before start of medication and after each treatment cycle.

Table 7.3 Side-effects

	Previously existing (%)	*First to third cycle* (%)	*Fourth to 18th cycle* (%)
Dysmenorrhoea			
slight	12.2	6.4	3.6
severe	4.2	0.5	0.2
Nausea	3.2	5.8	2.3
Vomiting	0.1	0.4	0.2
Dizziness	2.7	3.4	1.2
Breast tension	10.7	9.3	4.7
Headaches	10.1	8.6	6.1
migraine type	1.4	0.9	0.4
Nervousness	10.1	9.0	6.0
Depression	1.9	2.1	1.6
Increased libido	1.4	1.6	1.5
Decreased libido	2.9	4.5	3.3

To permit an overall view, the mean values of the percentile frequency of individual symptoms for the first to third medication cycles and for the 4th to 18th cycles were obtained and compared with pretreatment values (Table 7.3).

Although these subjective data must be evaluated with due reservation, it can be said that the test preparation is a very well tolerated, balanced drug both as regards side-effects ascribed to the oestrogen component as well as those ascribed to the progestagen component (see Table 7.3).

From the start of medication symptoms such as headache (including the migrainous type), nervousness and breast tension occur less frequently than in the pretreatment period. There is hardly any effect on libido. Serious thromboembolic disorders did not occur during the period of observation. Therapy was prematurely discontinued in 3 women because of the appearance of thrombophlebitis. One of these 3 women already had thrombophlebitis before treatment. Another case of thrombophlebitis that existed before the beginning of therapy and 2 more cases that arose during therapy were so slight that the physician in charge of the test did not regard them as contraindications or as a reason for discontinuing medication.

COMPARATIVE STUDY SH B 264 AB

Throughout the world the well-tolerated one-phase combination, containing 0.150 mg levonorgestrel and 0.03 mg ethinyloestradiol, belongs to the most widely used oral contraceptives. This product has undergone very intensive clinical investigation under the Code No. SH 7.1155. It attained this leading position in spite of the fact that the rate of intermenstrual bleeding – at least in the first few cycles of use – is definitely higher than that for preparations containing a daily dose of 0.05 mg of ethinyloestradiol. It was therefore of great interest to us to determine, in a comparative study, whether the new triphasic preparation offers a better cycle control than the fixed combination.

The planning design for this study required, for relevant differences between the two preparations, that a minimum of 200–250 women per trial group had to participate over a period of 6 cycles. The study was carried out in a randomized test arrangement in Great Britain, Sweden and Germany[5].

A total of 254 test persons received the triphasic SH B 264 AB for a total of 1440 cycles, while 236 women received the one-phase preparation SH 7.1155 for 1343 cycles. During these periods of observation no case of pregnancy occurred in any group. The tabular summary of the test results (Table 7.4) clearly indicates that, in fact, the triphasic contraceptive provides better cycle control than the fixed dose preparation.

Table 7.4 Clinical trial SH B 264 AB

	SH B 264 AB	*SH 7.1155*
Patients	254	236
Treatment cycles	1440	1343
Women who completed 6 cycles	226	211
Pregnancies	0	0
Breakthrough bleeding rate*	3.5%	4.7%
Spotting rate*	6.6%	11.0%
Amenorrhoea rate*	0.9%	2.3%

* As percentage of total number of treatment cycles

A very important advantage for the triphasic OC is its very low 'amenorrhoea rate'. This difference between the two preparations is statistically significant.

Table 7.4 further shows the differences in the incidence of spotting and breakthrough-bleeding. The differences in the

Table 7.5 Intermenstrual bleeding SH B 264 AB

	SH B 264 AB	*SH 7.1155*	
Cycle 1	15%	27%	$p<0.05$
Cycle 2	11%	21.5%	$p<0.05$

incidence of intermenstrual bleeding episodes are especially large in the first two medication cycles (Table 7.5); here they reach statistical significance at the $p<0.05$ level on the basis of

Fisher test calculations. Intermenstrual bleeding occurs more frequently when other low-oestrogen one-phase preparations are used[6] than with our 150/30 combination SH 7.1155 which occupies a very favourable positions among low-dose preparations as regards cycle control. Taking this into account, it becomes clear what a decisive improvement is brought about by the three-stage design of our triphasic trial preparation.

CONCLUSION

It can be deduced from both comparative studies that the triphasic test preparation SH B 264 AB which so far contains the lowest total steroid quantity of all available oral contraceptives wins on all counts:

(1) It offers reliable protection against conception.

(2) Tolerance and cycle control can only be designated as excellent. Though the progestagen dose was reduced by 40% from the 150/30 fixed combination level, the cycle control with the triphasic oral contraceptive is better than that of the reference preparation. The difference is most evident in the first two treatment cycles, which generally represent the 'critical phase' of low-dose medication. We hope that improved cycle control will increase the acceptability of low-dose oral contraception.

(3) The dose relations in the new product are in harmony with recent scientific knowledge concerning metabolic aspects of hormonal contraception.

References

1. Aydinlik, S., Lachnit, U. (1977). Diane-eine Gestagen-Östrogen-Kombination mit Antiandrogenwirkung. *Med. Mschr.*, **31**, 9, 425

2. Lachnit, U., Lehnert, J. (1973). Bericht über Phase III der klinischen Prüfung von Neogynon in Mitteleuropa. *Med. Mitt. Schering, Sonderdruck: Neogynon; Erfahrungen Untersuchungen*, Heft, Saldruck, Berlin 3
3. Lachnit, U. (1974). Bericht über die erweiterte klinische Prüfung eines neuen Zwei-Stufen-Präparates. *Ther. d. Gegenw.*, **113**, 1486
4. Lachnit, U. (1975). Einführung und weitere Ergebnisse zur klinischen Prüfung von Sequilar. *Med. Mitt. Schering*, **5**, 2
5. Zador, G. (1979). Fertility regulation using 'triphasic' administration of ethinylestradiol and levonorgestrel in comparison with the 30 plus 150 μg fixed dose regime. *Acta Obstet. Gynecol. Scand. Suppl.*, **88**
8. Alkemper, R., Rinz, Z. and Soergel, W. (1976). Clinical investigation of a very low dosage oral contraceptive combination: 0.75 mg lynestrenol and 0.0375 mg ethinyl oestradiol. *Curr. Med. Res. Opin.*, **4**, 353

8
Canadian experience with two triphasic oral contraceptive formulations

E. R. PLUNKETT, H. H. ALLEN and
R. PERCIVAL-SMITH

Most of the scientific community and the public recognize the importance of steroidal contraception and the improvements which have been made in their formulation. There is evidence that reduced dosage has been associated with a reduction of side-effects, including those of a more serious nature. At the same time, the prohibitive cost of new drug development, in time, manpower and economic terms, makes it essential to extract the maximum value from those steroids currently in use. Thus the search continues to produce a formulation which maintains efficacy and cycle control and which provides the least disruption of normal metabolic processes.

The progestagen norgestrel exists as levonorgestrel which is the biologically active enantiomer. The *dextro* form is considered to be inactive. Thus 100 μg of ($\pm$)-norgestrel would be equivalent in biological potency to 50 μg of the levonorgestrel. The WL-45 preparation described in this communication utilized ($\pm$)-norgestrel. However, for comparison purposes and to avoid confusion, all preparations described including WL-45 are expressed as levonorgestrel.

Exploring beyond the standard norgestrel-based compounds, Arnt *et al.*[1] compared three different levonorgestrel/ethinyloestradiol (EE) monophasic formulations; 150/20, 200/15 and 250/20. The two preparations containing 200 and 250 μg levonorgestrel were associated with better cycle control and appeared to be effective (no pregnancies reported in 537 and 562 cycles respectively).

Schneider *et al.*[2] studied two triphasic dosage formulations on a 6, 5, 10 day schedule. The levonorgestrel/EE content for SH B 264 AB was 30/50 (6 days), 40/75 (5 days) and 30/125 (10 days). The second preparation, SH B 261 AB was composed of 50/30, 50/50 and 125/40. A number of biochemical and biological responses were carefully studied. In effect, both preparations suppressed the LH surge and progesterone secretion, but the SH B 261 AB in the third treatment cycle failed to prevent mid-cycle rise of oestradiol-17β.

Selecting the SH B 264 AB formulation, Zador[3] has published a comparative study of this compound and the well established fixed dose combination of 150 μg and 30 μg levonorgestrel/EE. A total of 489 subjects was entered in the six-month project. Cycle control was better with the triphasic preparation and no pregnancies were reported by either group.

MATERIALS AND METHODS

To explore the feasibility of lowering the total oestrogen dose still further, a formulation designated as WL-45 was studied. Table 8.1 compares the three phase dosage schedule with WL-49(50), also referred to as SH B 264 AB. The EE content of WL-45 is less than that of WL-49(50) while the levonorgestrel levels are greater. It is perhaps of significance also to note the sequence of levonorgestrel doses is decreased from 200 μg in phase 1 to 150 in phase 2 in WL-45 while it progressively increases (50–75–125 μg) in the other preparation.

Table 8.1 Steroid content (μg of levonorgestrel/ethinyloestradiol) by treatment days

	Phase		
Triphasic	*1*	*2*	*3*
WL-45	200/15 (1–7)*	150/30 (8–14)	250/20 (15–21)
WL-49(50)	50/30 (1–6)	75/40 (7–11)	125/30 (12–21)

* Treatment days in parentheses

Table 8.2 Comparative total steroid content (μg per cycle) of four levonorgestrel oral contraceptives

	Levonorgestrel	*Ethinyloestradiol*
(1) 250/50 Monophasic	5250 (100%)*	1050 (100%)*
(2) 150/30 Monophasic	3150 (60%)*	630 (60%)*
WL-45	4200 (80%)* (133%)†	455 (43%)* (72%)†
WL-49(50)	1925 (36%* (60%)†	680 (64%)* (107%)†

* % of (1) † % of (2)

Table 8.2 compares the total steroidal content per cycle for the 2 standard monophasic compounds (250/50 and 150/30) and the 2 triphasic preparations under discussion. The progestagenic dominance of the WL-45 formulation and low oestrogen content is readily apparent.

Normal healthy volunteers were recruited, who exhibited no medical evidence which could be interpreted as being a contraindication to oral contraception. Ages ranged between 18 and 35 and about 50% had had at least one previous pregnancy. All were sexually active.

One investigator (H.H.A.) entered 69 cases studied through 624 cycles and the other (R.P.S.) entered 65 for 508 cycles. Thus a total of 134 subjects were observed over a maximum of 12 cycles for a total of 1132.

Blood lipids, including total cholestrol (TC) total triglycerides (TG), high density lipoprotein cholesterol (HDL-C) and the TC/HDL-C ratio are separated. The TCs and TGs were done in 2 centres and are described individually. The HDL-C and TC/HDL-C were done by one investigator only (H.H.A.). Subjects receiving WL-45 were studied prior to treatment and during the 6th and 12th cycles.

Preliminary blood lipid studies are also reported for time zero and during the 6th cycle for a group of women receiving the other triphasic formulation (WL-49(50)).

RESULTS

Effectiveness

No pregnancies have been reported for the combined series of 134 women treated for a total of 1132 cycles.

Table 8.3 Summary of missed menses and amenorrhoea by cycle (WL-45)

Cycle	*No. of patients*	*Missed menses*	%	*Amen-orrhoea*	%
1	134	4	2.9	0	0.0
2	131	10	7.6	1	0.7
3	119	6	5.0	0	2.4
4	112	2	1.7	2	7.0
5	105	6	5.7	3	9.5
6	100	4	4.0	7	8.0
7	88	3	3.4	5	6.8
8	78	0	0.0	3	7.6
9	75	8	10.6	2	2.6
10	68	2	2.9	2	3.0
11	63	4	6.3	3	4.8
12	59	2	3.3	3	5.2
Number of reports		51	4.5	31	4.6
Number of patients reporting		36	26.8	14	10.4

Cycle control

Missed menses and amenorrhoea

'Missed menses' is defined as failure to exhibit withdrawal bleeding in an isolated cycle as opposed to amenorrhoea which involves a failure to bleed for 2 or more consecutive cycles.

Table 8.4 Spotting and BTB by cycle (WL-45)

Cycle	*No. of patients*	*Spotting only*	%	*BTB only*	%	*Spotting and/or BTB*	%
1	134	27	20.1	47	35.0	84	62.6
2	131	20	15.2	31	23.6	60	45.8
3	119	11	9.2	22	18.4	38	31.9
4	112	12	10.7	23	20.5	41	36.6
5	105	12	11.4	17	16.1	33	31.4
6	100	10	10.0	19	19.0	34	34.0
7	88	11	12.5	12	13.6	26	29.5
8	78	6	7.6	13	16.6	23	29.4
9	75	6	8.0	14	18.6	23	30.6
10	68	2	2.9	6	8.8	8	11.7
11	63	5	7.9	5	7.9	11	17.4
12	59	3	5.0	8	13.5	11	18.6
Number of reports		125	11	217	19.1	392	34.6
Number of patients reporting		58	43.2	83	61.9	98	73.1

A total of 36 (26.8%) of the patients experienced at least one episode of missed menses. There were 51 reports in all (4.5% of 1132 cycles). Amenorrhoea was reported 47 times (4.1% of 1132 cycles) by 14 (10.4%) patients.

Table 8.3 indicates the numbers of reports by cycle and the numbers of continuing patients over the 12 cycles. It will be noted that the problem of missed menses and/or amenorrhoea occurred throughout the observation period with peaks most prominently seen in the first 7 or 8 cycles.

Spotting and breakthrough bleeding (BTB) (see Table 8.4)

There were 125 reports of spotting for an incidence of 11% of cycles. The incidence was 20.1% in the first cycle and continued to range between 9.2 and 12.5% between the 3rd and 7th. A total of 58 patients (43.2%) experienced the problem at least once.

Table 8.4 also provides the data for BTB and the combined figures for spotting and/or BTB. Forty-seven patients (35%) reported BTB in the first cycle and although there was some improvement subsequently, the incidence per cycle continued to range between 13.6 and 20.5 in cycles 3 to 9. There were a total of 217 reports or 19.1% of the 1132 cycles observed and 83 patients (61.9%) experienced this complication at least once.

Combining the data for spotting and/or BTB, there were 392 (34.6%) cycles in which one or both problems were reported. An overall total of 98 patients (73.1%) were involved.

Other side-effects

Tables 8.5 and 8.6 summarize the side-effects according to the ingredient to which they are generally attributed. Considering the subjective nature of most of the symptoms and the variations involved in eliciting and interpreting such information, there is surprising agreement between the two groups of data.

The mean body weight $\pm$ SEM for the combined groups was 134.78 $\pm$ 5.18 lbs initially, compared with 135.26 $\pm$ 5.13 lbs and 135.49 $\pm$ 5.17 lbs at 6 and 12 months respectively. Though the increments were small, they were significant ($p < 0.05$).

The blood pressure did not exhibit a consistent change between the initial determinations when compared with the values obtained during the 6th and 12th cycles. The systolic pressures were 118 $\pm$ 2.0, 123 $\pm$ 2.2 and 119 $\pm$ 2.3 at the three intervals, while the diastolic readings were 73 $\pm$ 1.6, 74 $\pm$ 1.4 and 73 $\pm$ 1.6 respectively.

Table 8.5 Oestrogen related side-effects for WL-45

	Allen				*Percival-Smith*			
	patients		*cycles*		*patients*		*cycles*	
	No.	%	*No.*	%	*No.*	%	*No.*	%
G.I. symptoms	0	0.0	0	0.0	1	1.5	1	0.2
Abdominal cramps	22*	31.9	57	9.1	33*	50.8	74	14.6
Leg cramps	4*	5.8	7	1.1	8	12.3	9	1.8
Migraine headaches	2*	2.9	3	0.5	0	0	0	0
Simple headache	16*	23.2	45	7.2	22	33.9	56	11.0
Nausea	9	13.0	32	5.1	19	29.2	32	6.3
Bloating/oedema	7	10.1	15	2.4	8	12.3	20	3.9
Vaginal infections	2*	2.9	2	0.3	1*	1.5	1	0.2
Vaginal discharge	7*	10.1	13	2.1	11*	16.9	30	5.9
Sore breasts	6*	8.7	16	2.6	6*	9.2	19	3.7
Irritability	3*	4.4	6	1.0	8*	12.3	18	3.5
Chloasma	2	2.9	2	0.3	0	0.0	0	0.0
No. of patients/cycles studied	69/624				65/508			

* These symptoms are more common during 3 pre-treatment cycles (by history)

Table 8.6 Progestagen related side-effects for WL-45

	Allen				*Percival-Smith*			
	patients		*cycles*		*patients*		*cycles*	
	No.	%	*No.*	%	*No.*	%	*No.*	%
Acne	5*	7.3	9	1.4	6*	9.2	22	4.3
Appetite increase	2*	2.9	4	0.6	3*	4.6	4	0.8
Depression	6*	8.7	11	1.7	7*	10.8	12	1.9
Fatigue	4*	5.8	14	2.2	7*	10.8	11	1.7
Decreased libido	3	4.4	7	1.1	1	1.5	4	0.8
Increase in breast size	1*	1.5	1	0.2	3*	4.6	15	3.0
Weight gain	2	2.9	3	0.5	1	1.5	1	0.2
Vaginal dryness	3	4.4	4	0.6	5	7.7	16	3.2
No. of patients/cycles studied	69/624				65/508			

* These symptoms are more common during 3 pre-treatment cycles (by history)

Lipid profiles

Table 8.7 summarizes the available lipid data from the two reporting centres. WL-45 appeared to exert no significant effect on the cholesterol or triglycerides at 6 and 12 months when compared to the pretreatment control. Similarly, no significant change was noted at 6 months with the WL-49(50) triphasic preparation.

The HDL cholesterol rose significantly ($p < 0.01$) between 6 and 12 months in the WL-45 treated patients and decreased slightly but not significantly in the first 6 cycles of WL-49(50) treatment.

The TC/HDL-C ratio dropped significantly ($p < 0.05$) between the 6th and 12th cycles of WL-45 therapy while a very small but significant ($p < 0.05$) increment occurred in the first 6 cycles of WL-49(50) use.

DISCUSSION

Obviously cycle control is a major problem in patients taking WL-45. The rate of missed menses and/or amenorrhoea and BTB or spotting effectively eliminates this formulation as an acceptable oral contraceptive.

The progestagen dominance associated with a very low oestrogen content could account readily for the amenorrhoea and/or missed menses. The spotting and/or BTB might be explained on the basis of the generally low estrogen content. On the other hand between phases 1 and 2, the WL-45 formulation decreases the levonorgestrel content from 200 to 150 μg. The number of cycles reporting spotting and/or BTB during the 2nd phase of administration was 79 as opposed to 25 in the 1st phase and 51 in the third. In contrast, WL-49(50) which is associated with excellent cycle control, is formulated on the basis of a stepwise increase in levonorgestrel (50, 75 and 125 μg).

Although the effectiveness of WL-45 appears to be excellent

Table 8.7 Lipoprotein values for WL-45/49(50) studies (means ± standard errors)

Triphasic (investigator)	*Sample size*	*Cycle No.*	*Total cholesterol*[a] *(TC)*	*Triglycerides*[b]	*HDL-cholesterol*[c] *(HDL-C)*	*Ratio TC/HDL-C*
WL-45	25	0	170.8 ± 7.7	87.8 ± 13.0	—	—
(Percival-		6	165.8 ± 7.1	84.3 ± 9.0	—	—
Smith)		12	178.0 ± 7.3	75.9 ± 7.6	—	—
WL-45	10	0	201.0 ± 9.2	85.8 ± 8.6	47.9 ± 4.3	4.4 ± 0.3
(Allen)		6	209.4 ± 8.7	92.6 ± 8.6	46.7 ± 2.4**	4.6 ± 0.3***
		12	209.8 ± 8.6	89.5 ± 12.7	52.5 ± 3.3**	4.1 ± 0.3***
WL-49(50)	24	0	208.0 ± 6.7	103.0 ± 13.6	55.6 ± 2.3	3.9 ± 0.2*
(Allen)		6	210.0 ± 8.5	114.0 ± 14.4	52.8 ± 2.4	4.1 ± 0.2*

Reference ranges (mg/100 ml): [a] 150–260 (Percival-Smith), 135–300 (Allen). [b] 10–180 (Percival-Smith), 30–160 (Allen). [c] 30–70 (Allen).

* $p < 0.05$ for increase. ** $p < 0.01$ for increase. *** $p < 0.05$ for decrease.

and the lack of any adverse effect upon the lipid factors examined is appealing, the preparation is unsuitable for the reasons noted above.

Further study of the WL-45 preparation has been discontinued in favour of WL-49(50) which combines a low total oestrogen and low progestagen content. Our experience with this latter triphasic formulation, like that of others, has been very favourable.

References

1. Arnt, I. C., Ferrari, A., Sartoretto, J. N. and Woutersz, T. D. (1977). *Fertil. Steril.*, **28**, 549
2. Schneider, W. H. F., Spona, J., Schmid, R. and Lachnit-Fixson, U. (1977). In Haspels, A. A. and Kay, C. R. (eds.), *International Symposium on Hormonal Contraception*. (Amsterdam: Excerpta Medica)
3. Zador, G. (1979). *Acta Obstet. Gynaecol. Scand. Suppl.*, **88**, 43

Discussion

Editor's note: The following questions and answers have been selected from the transcript of the discussion. They form a representative cross-section of the discussion but are not a complete record.

Question: What data are available on acne and the new triphasic pill?

Answer: During the clinical investigation acne cleared up in 22 out of 26 women who suffered from acne at the beginning of the trial within the first year of treatment. This nice 'side-effect' probably results from the considerable reduction of the progestagen content in the triphasic preparation. The low progestagen content hardly exerts any residual androgenic effect whereas endogenic androgen synthesis is decreased by inhibition of ovulation and SHBG is increased by the oestrogen component of our preparation.

Question: Do percentages of spotting and breakthrough bleeding differ from cycle to cycle?

Answer: Spotting and BTB occur more frequently at the beginning of medication; with increasing duration of treatment the bleeding rates drop continuously, for BTB down to zero at the end of the first year of medication.

Questions: (1) What clinical studies have been done on women in the third world? Are the suggested low doses suitable for women with problems such as malabsorption?

(2) What pregnancy rates have you had in the 'developed' countries versus the third world?

Answers: (1) The extended clinical study was a multicentred one including Peru and Venezuela. We have seen the same contraceptive efficacy in these countries as in European countries and the same low rates of side-effects. Special studies in women with malabsorption syndrome have not been conducted. To my knowledge studies of this kind are presently being carried out by WHO with different oral contraceptives.

(2) Up to now we have evaluated 10 000 documented treatment cycles for contraceptive reliability. In these documented cycles we had no pregnancies; neither in Europe nor in the so-called third world. One pregnancy has been reported from Venezuela, but this pregnancy is most probably a patient- and not a method failure (omission of tablets with frequent bleeding episodes and intake of a strong laxative during OC medication).

Question: The biphasic oral contraceptive mimics the normal menstrual cycle and this is supposed to be an advantage. However, is this also true for patients with breast tension, dysmenorrhoea and endometriosis?

Answer: Our data show that the triphasic contraceptive exerts a beneficial influence on breast tension and dysmenorrhoea: both symptoms occur less frequently under treatment than in the control period before the start of the trial. In patients suffering from endometriosis who wish to take an oral contraceptive, we recommend a progestagen-dominant fixed dose preparation. We think that the low dose triphasic OC is not suitable for these women.

Question: Is there any *definite* clinical evidence that using less than 50 μg of ethinyloestradiol reduces thromboembolic complications?

Answer: I see Dr Wiseman is in the audience. Since he has done some work on this topic, it might be useful if he were to answer the question.

Dr Wiseman: The question presupposes that there is a cause–effect relationship between oral contraceptives and thromboembolic complications, and I would argue that the evidence for such an association is very tenuous. Professor Greenblatt in his Introduction touched on the results of the RCGP paper[1] and the fact that the *total* number of deaths in Pill-users and in controls was fairly similar; he might have added that the preponderance of deaths from circulatory disease in Pill-users in that study was made up of nine deaths from subarachnoid haemorrhage, which is paradoxical since that is not a thrombotic disease.

Two interesting papers appeared recently in the *Lancet* and the *British Medical Journal*; one, by Meade and his colleagues[2], suggested that there was a risk of arterial disease, and that this risk was associated with the progestagen component of the combined oral contraceptive. They concluded that the lower the dose of progestagen the less the risk. If this were true, then clearly the amount of oestrogen would not be relevant. In the other paper, Bottiger *et al.*[3] from Sweden examined the incidence of arterial disease during a time when oestrogen dosage in the Pill was low and stated that there was a significant decrease in the incidence of venous thromboembolic disease as compared to an earlier time when the dosage was high, but that there was no significant change in arterial disease. Thus it seems that the conclusions of these two papers are contradictory.

I have recently looked at this question of circulatory disease from the point of view of the incidence of such disease in the total population of the United Kingdom[4]. I found that between the years 1962 and 1976 deaths from circulatory disease in women of reproductive age fell steadily from 32.9 per 100 000 population to 21.7 per 100 000 population. This decrease did not occur in older women and the decrease in young women was greater than in men of comparable age. During this period, oral contraceptives, which were introduced in 1961, rose steadily in sales to a peak of 45 000 000 in 1976. It is not logical with these data to hypothesize that oral contraceptives during a period of high and increasing usage cause diseases which during the same period have been falling steadily. Indeed, a case could be made out that OCs are protective against circulatory disease. At the very least, these results are opposed to the results of many prospective or retrospective investigations, and serious doubt must therefore be cast on the conclusions of those other studies about a causal relationship between OCs and thromboembolism.

That said, it is nevertheless sensible on general medical grounds to prescribe an oral contraceptive – or any other treatment, for that matter – with the lowest dose which is compatible with maximal reliability and acceptability.

Question: Is there any increase in fibrocystic disease of the breast with the triphasic preparation?

Answer: The experiences with the triphasic oral contraceptive are no different than with the standard oral contraceptives in use. According to Fechner the incidence of benign breast disease has been found to be less in women on oestrogen–progestagen preparations than in non-Pill takers. In fact, many clinicians have successfully employed the combination pill in the management of mastodynia and mazoplasia. In studies with the triphasic preparation it appears that the incidence of breast tenderness was reduced.

Question: How does the triphasic compare with the standard oral contraceptives which are alleged to increase thromboembolic disease (thrombophlebitis, myocardial infarction, cerebral thrombosis) because they increase coagulation factors?

Answer: The changes in coagulation factors while on oral contraceptives are no different from those seen in normal pregnancy. Actually, antithrombin III activity is altered less while on the triphasic than with other oral contraceptives. Thromboembolic disease is seen far more frequently in women on oral contraceptives who smoke. The choice is theirs: not to smoke if they wish to enjoy the security of the Pill. Furthermore, these untoward effects are seen more frequently in women who have a history of heart disease and/or toxaemia of pregnancy and are over 35 years of age. Although oral contraceptives are not recommended for women over 35, the triphasic preparation may be used because of its mildness, and the fact that it does not have any untoward effect on HDL levels. The woman over 35 needs protection against conception more than the younger woman because of increased morbidity and mortality associated with pregnancy in the older age group and the increased risk of chromosomal defects in the offspring of mothers. The triphasic pill may be recommended to women over 35 to whom the risk of hormonal conception control is adequately explained, who do not smoke, and who do not have a history of heart or cardiovascular disease.

Question: How do the parameters of metabolic change in the classic Pill compare with those of the triphasic?

Answer: It is difficult to make comparisons unless the populations studied are large, have similar diets, are subjected more or less to similar stresses, etc. It should be recalled that different oral contraceptives have different oestrogen contents and the progestagen content differs in potency and chemical design. Some progestagens are androgenic, others are more progestagenic; some, in fact, are anti-oestrogenic, others are slightly oestrogenic. Some factors, for instance, may have some bearing on levels of triglycerides and high density lipoprotein cholesterol (HDL-cholesterol). In general, oral contraceptives increase triglycerides and reduce high density lipoproteins. Although the triphasic oral contraceptive in question raised triglycerides, it had none of the unwanted effects on HDL-cholesterol. It may be said that, in general, oral contraceptives with low oestrogen and a high amount of progestagens have the tendency to reduce HDL. In this context, then, the low dose levonorgestrel found in the triphasic Pill is advantageous.

References

1. Royal College of General Practitioners (1977). *Lancet*, **2**, 727
2. Meade, T. W., Greenberg, G. and Thompson, S. G. (1980). *Br. Med. J.*, **280**, 1157
3. Bottiger, L. E., Boman, G., Eklund, G. and Westerholm, B. (1980). *Lancet*, **1**, 8178
4. Wiseman, R. A. and MacRae, K. D. (to be published)

Summary

R. B. GREENBLATT

The original oral contraceptives contained more oestrogen in the form of ethinyloestradiol or mestranol and progestagen in the form of norethynodrel or norethisterone than was necessary for conception control. There has been a trend over the years to reduce dosages of both components in order to minimize side-effects while ensuring effectiveness. However, as dosages were lowered, there has been an increase in spotting and break-through bleeding during the first few months of their administration.

The sequential pill appeared more physiological in that it followed more closely physiological principles, but the need to employ large doses of EE or EE3ME to inhibit ovulation and the higher pregnancy rate made the sequential regimen less attractive or useful.

A triphasic formulation has become available that takes advantage of the synergism between ethinyloestradiol and the potent levonorgestrel so that low doses of the oestrogen and very low doses of the progestagen could be employed with great effectiveness. Such a preparation is relatively free from side-effects, partly because the basic pharmacological tenet of the minimal dose for the desired result and the division of the cycle into three parts using 30 μg of EE for the first 6 days, then 5 days of 40 μg, followed by 30 μg for 10 days, for a total of 21 days, thus more or less mimicking the physiological rise and fall of oestrogens during the normal cycle. The amount of EE used in the cycle, which alone would not inhibit ovulation consistently, totals 680 μg for the 21 days and compares very favourably with the 630 μg of EE now used in the lowest dosage oestrogen-progestagen contraceptive pill. Oestrogens favourably increase HDL. The progestagen used in the triphasic pill follows the pattern of gradual increasing dosages, i.e. 50 μg for 6 days, 75 μg for 5 days and 125 μg for the last 10 days, for a total of 1925 μg for 21 days. Compare this total dosage of the progestagen with the dose employed in the most commonly used 'low dose pills', i.e. 10 500 μg of norgestrel or 21 000 μg of norethindrone, or 21 000 μg of ethynodiol diacetate. The incidence of hypertension has recently been shown to be related to the magnitude of the progestagen employed. Furthermore, the more androgenic the pill and the greater the dosage, the greater the untoward effect of lowering HDL.

Because the low dose EE and low dose levonorgestrel in the new triphasic regimen show excellent suppression of pituitary ovarian action and maintain a cervical mucus that is hostile to sperm migration, there is almost totally effective conception control. Furthermore, such a formulation does not appear to jeopardize rapid return of ovulation on withdrawal. The triphasic pill should be regarded as an important advance in conception control.

Dr Michael Briggs, from Australia, compared the triphasic presentation with other combined oral contraceptives. He concluded that, while unwanted changes in lipid, carbohydrate, and lipoprotein factors, together with disturbances in coagulation factors and the renin–angiotensin system, are seen with higher-dose formulations, they are minimal with the new triphasic formulation, WL-49(50) (SH B 264 AB).

Dr Ulf Larsson-Cohn, from Sweden, believes that in order to get a meaningful interpretation of the lipid effects of a therapeutic agent one must measure more than just plasma concentrations of cholesterol and triglycerides. He presented results of studies involving a number of combinations of LNg and EE and the new triphasic pill and their effects on SHBG and lipid metabolism. In conclusion he said that too much emphasis has been given to the oestrogen component and that the significance of the progestagen has been neglected. In designing an oral contraceptive, it is important to weigh the negative and positive effects of both.

Dr Virginia Upton, from the United States, discussed the physiological basis for the triphasic approach and the viewpoint that such an approach should lessen systemic side-effects by virtue of rescheduled and lower steroid content of the formulation, and lessen interference with normal hypothalamic–pituitary function, without compromising contraceptive effectiveness. The new triphasic formulation, WL-49(50) (SH B 264 AB), was discussed in the light of these mechanisms and contrasted with more traditional formulations.

Dr Jurgen Spona, from Austria, investigated the ovulation-inhibiting dose of oral levonorgestrel to find appropriate doses for new formulations and the mode of action of triphasic oral contraception. His observations suggest that the new triphasic oral contraceptive SH B 264 AB (WL-49(50)) acts by inhibiting ovulation and by providing a back-up mechanism by reducing the cervical score. The reduction of levonorgestrel dose in the new triphasic does not interfere with cycle control, since the triphasic oral contraceptive mimics endogenous sex hormone patterns of the normal cycle.

Dr Ursula Lachnit-Fixson, from West Germany, discussed the rationale for the new triphasic oral contraceptive and reviewed the progress made over the years in reducing the dose of both components. This culminated in the triphasic preparation containing the lowest possible quantity of both hormone components, with oestrogen doses in mid-cycle fitting in with the normal pre-ovulatory peak. Even the first pilot studies showed that such an arrangement, when compared to other low-dose preparations, resulted in clearly improved cycle control. Dr Lachnit later presented and discussed the results of two successful extended comparative trials.

Dr Earl Plunkett, from Canada, described a preliminary study undertaken to explore the potential of two triphasic oral contraceptives. The investigation resulted in a preference for the formulation of the new triphasic WL-49(50) (SH B 264 AB).

Dr Robert Greenblatt, of the United States, believes that the woman over 35 needs to be protected against conception even more so than the younger woman and therefore should not be denied the new low-dose triphasic contraceptive agent despite the fact that several agencies feel that oral contraceptives are contraindicated in the woman over 35.